NURSING ASSESSMENT

WILEY NURSING CONCEPT MODULE

Series Editor:
FAY L. BOWER, R.N., M.S.N.
Professor of Nursing
San Jose State University
San Jose, California

NURSING ASSESSMENT

Consultant:
Robinetta Wheeler, R.N., M.S.
Doctoral Student
Department of Behavioral
and Social Sciences
School of Nursing
University of California, San Francisco

A WILEY MEDICAL PUBLICATION
JOHN WILEY & SONS
New York • London • Sydney • Toronto

Wiley Nursing Concept Modules

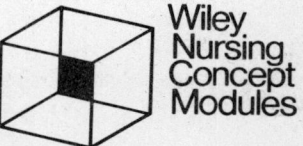

Copyright © 1977 by John Wiley & Sons, Inc.

All rights reserved. Published simultaneously in Canada.

No part of this book may be reproduced by any means, nor transmitted, nor translated into a machine language without the written permission of the publisher.

Library of Congress Cataloging in Publication Data:

Main entry under title:

Nursing assessment.

   (Wiley nursing concept module) (A Wiley medical publication)
   1. Nursing. 2. Diagnosis. I. Wheeler, Robinetta. II. Series. [DNLM: 1. Nursing—Programmed texts. WY18 N9755]
RT48.N87   610.73   77-5160
ISBN 0-471-02167-9

Printed in the United States of America

10 9 8 7 6 5 4 3 2 1

CONTRIBUTORS

Toni Heilman, R.N., M.S.
Instructor
College of Nursing
The University of Arizona
Tucson, Arizona

Lois M. Hoskins, R.N., M.S.
Assistant Professor
School of Nursing
Catholic University of America
Washington, D.C.

Suzanne Hall Johnson, R.N., M.N.
Formerly, Instructor
Department of Nursing
San Jose State University
San Jose, California

Ralph Matteoli, R.N., M.S.
Associate Professor
Department of Nursing
San Francisco State University
San Francisco, California

Gloria C. Schmidt, R.N., M.N.
Formerly, Assistant Professor
College of Nursing
Arizona State University
Tempe, Arizona

Robinetta Wheeler, R.N., M.S.
Doctoral Student
Department of Behavioral
and Social Sciences
School of Nursing
University of California, San Francisco

Staff Nurse
Veterans Administration Hospital
Palo Alto, California

SERIES PREFACE

During the last decade there have been major changes in instructional formats. In an attempt to provide learning experiences that meet individual needs and abilities, educators have tried various instructional methods such as audiotutorial learning, independent study, and most recently, learning modules. Students of all ages, studying a wide variety of subjects, have been introduced to modular programs.

Of all the new instructional approaches, learning modules have taken the lead. Administrators and teachers feel encouraged about them because they permit the implementation of learning principles. Their popularity is also partly due to their flexibility for learner use and their economic use of teacher time. Teachers employing modules can spend time with the slower learners while the faster learners proceed on their own.

The term *module* did not originate in the field of education. The term has various meanings—components of television sets, parts of a spacecraft, construction units of a building. In education *module* refers to a self-contained package dealing with a single conceptual entity that can be completed at a time and place determined by the learner.

This volume is a collection of learning modules about a specific subject. Each module in the book deals with a portion of the subject and follows the same format: pretest, learning objectives, directions, activities, progress checks, and posttest. The modules are designed for independent learner use, but they can also be used as a basis for seminars. Some of the learning modules refer the learner to media—tapes, films, slides, books, or games. All the modules suggest learning activities.

This volume of modules can be used in schools of nursing by students and teachers and by nurses in staff development programs. They were designed to fit into any curriculum pattern and any staff development program.

Praise and thanks are due the authors of the modules, who have prepared them from expert knowledge of the content and from a desire to make learning enjoyable and rewarding. Special thanks to the many students, too many to list here, who have encouraged me to publish modules for their use. Their suggestions, critiques, and encouragement have made this book a reality.

Fay L. Bower

CONTENTS

INTRODUCTION TO NURSING ASSESSMENT 1
Robinetta Wheeler

THE NURSING HISTORY 25
Toni Heilman

PHYSICAL HEALTH ASSESSMENT 57
Gloria C. Schmidt

PSYCHOSOCIAL ASSESSMENT 87
Ralph Matteoli, Part 1
Robinetta Wheeler, Part 2

THE NURSING DIAGNOSIS 119
Lois M. Hoskins

THE EVALUATION PROCESS 143
Suzanne Hall Johnson

NURSING ASSESSMENT

ROBINETTA WHEELER, R.N., M.S.

WILEY NURSING CONCEPT MODULE

INTRODUCTION TO NURSING ASSESSMENT

CONTENTS
- **PRETEST 3**   Answers 5
- **INTRODUCTION 6**
- **TERMINAL OBJECTIVES 6**
   - ACTIVITY 1.   Assessment: A Definition   7
   - ACTIVITY 2.   Areas Essential to an Adequate Health Assessment   9
   - ACTIVITY 3.   Making an Assessment   11
- **POSTTEST 20**   Answers 22
- **REFERENCES 23**

© 1977 Wiley

PRETEST

1. Define the word assessment:

2. Describe the difference between the following words and assessment:
   a. judgment

   b. evaluation

   c. interpretation

   d. diagnosis

3. The steps in the process of making an assessment are:
   Circle the number with the correct answers.
   a. read client's chart   1. a, b, and d
   b. sort and categorize data   2. c, b, and d
   c. select area to be assessed   3. b only
   d. write assessment statement   4. all of these
   e. gather data   5. b, c, d, e

4. In the examples below, identify the method used to gather data.
   a. Dr. Maria Sonia invited Mrs. Perry to her office. She asked Mrs. Perry to describe the layout of their home. She explained that Mr. Perry's leg would be in a cast for two more months.
      The method used is _____.
   b. John Starp is a student nurse. He has begun clinical experience in a well baby clinic. He finds that many of the mothers say they have been there before. He plans to read the clinical record of each client the day before the client's visit.
      The method used is _____.
   c. Josie has been watching the children play with the dolls through a one-way mirror. She learned a lot about the feelings children often experience and do not express.
      The method used is _____.
   d. Mr. Warner has just found out that he has to have a proctoscopy. He goes to his local library and borrows a book on the subject.
      The method used is _____.

5. Match the word with the correct description.
   ____1. published articles on a subject; books   a. interview
   ____2. accounts of past events   b. records
   ____3. a directed question-and-answer ses-   c. observation
          sion between two or more people   d. literature
   ____4. the result of using one of the five sen-
          ses or the result of an experiment; a
          measurement

© 1977 Wiley

4 NURSING ASSESSMENT

6. A criterion for a physician to legally practice medicine is a current license from the state in which he practices. Which of the following methods would you use to gather the most accurate data about a physician's license? Circle the correct answer(s).
   a. observation
   b. records
   c. interview
   d. literature

7. You do not know the criteria for performing a mental-status exam. You do which of the following? Circle the correct answer(s).
   a. ask a psychiatrist
   b. assist in performing one
   c. read a psychology text
   d. listen to a tape on the psychiatric evaluation

8. Read the following situation, then identify at least five categories for sorting the data.

   Peter Rawn is a 40-year-old black man. He has been hospitalized for a myocardial infarction. The doctor plans to discharge him in two days. Mr. Rawn is married with three children. He describes his wife as an active woman of 38 years. His children are in high school. Mr. Rawn is employed as an assistant principal in the local junior high school. He has had hypertension since the age of 35. The doctor has informed him that he must lose weight and decrease his activities. He plays golf regularly. Mr. Rawn's father died from a heart attack. Mr. Rawn tells the nurse that he knows he has to do what the doctor suggests. "However, it's so hard to eat differently from the rest of the family. Plus my job demands that I take visitors out for lunch. How can I diet and meet my job responsibilities? I also need to work. I plan for all my children to go to college."

9. Sort the data in question 8 under the categories identified.

10. Write an assessment statement for the data sorted in question 9.

11. The term holism means that the whole health-care team plans care. Circle the correct answer.   True   False

12. An explanation for the multidimensional nursing assessment must include the following. Circle the correct answer(s).
    a. describe today's trends
    b. refer to the changing character of man

© 1977 Wiley

c. speak to the simplistic model of man
d. examine the concept of holism

13. The first priority for man's safety is a threat to life. Circle the correct answer.   True   False

14. The second priority for man's safety is a threat to his normal growth and development. Circle the correct answer.   True   False

15. The third priority for man's safety is the threat of destructive change. Circle the correct answer.   True   False

Answers

1. The process of gathering data, sorting and categorizing them, and making a summary statement.

2. a. judgment: differs from assessment in that it compares theoretical and practical data, then makes an opinion statement about the data.
   b. evaluation: concerns only a comparison to determine worth.
   c. interpretation: explanation of meaning of data.
   d. diagnosis: uses results from assessment, judgment, then makes interpretation as it relates to pathology.

3. 5

4. a. interview
   b. records
   c. observation
   d. literature

5. 1. d
   2. b
   3. a
   4. c

6. Circle b—Records (contacting State Department). a—Observation would be possible if license were displayed in physician's office.

7. Circle all.

8. Possible categories: present condition, family situation, employment status, health history, culture, aspirations, interests, spirituality.

9.

Family Situation	Present Condition	Employment Status
Married	Recovering from myocardial infarct	Assistant principal
Three children—all in high school	Hypertensive	Often takes visitors out for lunch
Wife 38 years old, active woman	Overweight	
	Thinks it's difficult to eat differently than others	

Health History	Culture	Interests
Father died of heart attack	Black American	Plays golf
Developed hypertension at 35 years of age		

© 1977 Wiley

Spirituality	*Aspirations*
No data	Wants all children to attend college
	Wants to work

10. Mr. Rawn is a 40-year-old black American recovering from myocardial infarct. He must lose weight and decrease his activities. He is concerned about continuing his job, sending his children to college, and difficulty of dieting.
11. False
12. b and d
13. True
14. False
15. False

INTRODUCTION

Assessment as a part of the nursing process has been receiving a lot of attention in the nursing literature. This seems to imply that nurses are doing something new. Actually nurses have always been making assessments. The recent trend merely recognizes and focuses on this part of the nursing process.

Making assessments is not unique to nursing or only to health workers. Assessments are made daily by every human being on a variety of subjects. This module will introduce the reader to the process of making an assessment in nursing. Terms will be defined in Activity 1. Activity 2 will present the steps in the process. Finally, Activity 3 will discuss the areas essential to an adequate health assessment.

This is an introductory module in a volume on the assessment process in nursing. This volume contains modules on taking a nursing history, making a psychosocial assessment, the physical health assessment, the nursing diagnosis, and the evaluation process.

TERMINAL OBJECTIVES

At the completion of this module, the learner will be able to:

1. define the word assessment
2. describe the difference between assessment and judgment, evaluation, interpretation, and diagnosis
3. identify the steps in the assessment process
4. describe the methods of data collection
5. given an example, identify the method used for data collection
6. given criteria, select an appropriate method for data collection
7. given data, sort and categorize them
8. given an example, demonstrate the ability to make a nursing-assessment summary statement
9. define the term holism

© 1977 Wiley

10. explain reasons for the multidimensional nursing assessment approach
11. given the threats for humans, their families or communities, order them for priority

ACTIVITY 1
ASSESSMENT: A DEFINITION

When one hears the word assessment, any number of definitions may come to mind. Some synonyms often given for assessment are judgment, evaluation, interpretation, and diagnosis.

A dictionary definition of *assessment* is "... setting an estimated value on property, etc. for taxation or for determination of damages."[1]

A definition given for *judgment* is "... the ability to come to an opinion of things; power of comparing and deciding...."[2]

An *evaluation* is defined as "... determining the value or amount of; an appraisal."[3]

An *interpretation* is defined as "... an explanation of the meaning...."[4]

A *diagnosis* is defined as "... the act or process of deciding the nature of a diseased condition by examination."[5]

It is evident that these words have overlapping meanings. The nursing literature is equally confusing.

Wolanin notes that the word assessment has been used to describe parts of the nursing process other than the data-gathering part. She defines assessment as "... the process of observing and gathering data."[6]

Lewis describes assessment as "... the collection of data about the patient from a variety of sources and the categorization of these data into problem areas."[7]

Bower[8] lists the requirements of assessment as:

1. extracting relevant facts and concepts from the situation
2. classifying and sorting these data into groups that demonstrate relationships
3. making interpretations of the situation based on the interrelatedness of these groupings

The use of the term assessment in nursing literature may or may not include the judgment component. The term evaluation also contains a judgment component. In the nursing literature, the importance of evaluation centers around effectiveness of nursing interventions. As interpretation of the meaning of data is considered a part of the nursing process. The conflict seems to be whether or not it is a part of the assessment. Diagnosis presents a similar problem, as by definition it necessitates an interpretation.

Bloch explores the various definitions and uses of a number of terms in nursing, including assessment. She suggests that assessment in nursing be defined as having two separate processes—data collection and problem identification.[9]

Doona developed a theory of judgment in nursing. She describes judgment in nursing as "interaction between nursing concepts and nursing facts. The judgment evolves from the refinement process of the concepts acting on facts and the facts acting on concepts."[10]

[1, 2, 3, 4, 5] *Webster's New World Dictionary*, 1964.

[6] Wolanin, Mary Opal, "Nursing Assessment," 1976.

[7] Lewis, Lucille, *Planning Patient Care*, 1970.

[8] Bower, Fay Louise, *The Process of Planning Nursing Care: A Practice Model*, 1976.

[9] Bloch, Doris, "Some Crucial Terms in Nursing—What Do They Really Mean?" 1974.

[10] Doona, Mary Ellen, "The Judgment Process in Nursing," 1976.

© 1977 Wiley

Nursing needs clarity on these definitions. For purposes of this module the definitions are:

assessment: the process of gathering data, sorting and categorizing them, and making a summary statement.

judgment: the result of comparing data and forming an opinion about their relationship to each other. Includes use of theoretical and practical data.

evaluation: the result of comparing data for the purpose of deciding worth.

interpretation: the explanation of the meaning of data.

diagnosis: the interpretive statement made at the completion of an assessment and judgment and related to pathology.

This author suggests the removal of judgment from the definition of assessment, since it involves another step. An assessment should present what *is*. A judgment can then be made about what is, applying principles and theories to the assessment data. The interpretation of assessment and judgment in terms of disease and problems is made in the diagnosis. The term evaluation should be reserved for use after an intervention has occurred, since it tests only for value that is dependent on social context.

EXAMPLE

A psychologist administers a series of tests to an individual. She is making an assessment, i.e., gathering data. The scores tell her about the tasks the testee can perform. She compares the scores of one test with the norms for that test, then compares the various test scores to each other. Next she makes a judgment, i.e., she forms an opinion based on the correlation between scores. Her next step is to describe the meaning of her judgment, which is an interpretation. The diagnosis is interpretation of the assessment and judgment in terms of the categories of psychological pathology. Then the psychologist can suggest interventions, such as practicing certain skills or using certain techniques. Once these interventions have been accomplished, evaluations can be made regarding their effectiveness.

PROGRESS CHECK

Match the following:

___1. comparing data for determination of worth

___2. an interpretive statement about an assessment and judgment, related to pathology

___3. an explanation of the meaning of data

___4. gathering data, sorting and categorizing them; includes a summary statement

___5. comparison of data leading to an opinion of relationship

a. diagnosis
b. judgment
c. evaluation
d. assessment
e. interpretation

ANSWERS
1. c
2. a
3. e
4. d
5. b

© 1977 Wiley

ACTIVITY 2
AREAS ESSENTIAL TO AN ADEQUATE HEALTH ASSESSMENT

Philosophers have discussed and debated human nature for centuries. A human being has been viewed as only a body, as a body and a mind, and more recently as a physical, mental, and social being. Still there is something missed. The essence of a human being is more than a triad.

The term holism refers to the view of a person as a total being more than the sum of his or her parts. Rogers[11] describes the human as an open system continually interacting with his or her environment. Owing to this interaction, a person, at any point in time, is the product of all that has preceded him or her to that time. Homeodynamics describes the continual interaction process between a human and his or her world. Since life is unidirectional and a person is an open system, he or she will continue to change as he or she moves through life. Therefore one cannot understand a person out of the context of his or her position in time and space—hence the need for nursing to go beyond the diad or triad models of the human being.

When making an assessment of a client, one must observe many aspects besides physical condition. Activity 3 will develop categories for sorting data. The lists are incomplete. When working with the client the nurse needs to continually change the repetoire of categories. There needs to be flexibility to allow as much expansion as necessary to obtain a total assessment of the client. This is a process; it does not occur from a one-time intervention.

In practice the number of client-nurse contacts may be limited. This makes it crucial that the nurse approach a client as a total being from the first contact. Interventions will be ineffectual unless the client's culture, spiritual, intellectual, and social needs are considered. Many nurses can think of incidents where clients did not follow through with a prescribed treatment. Perhaps in such cases the assessment was incomplete or merely physical.

Nursing is becoming more aware of the variations in people and their needs. The area of death and dying, too, has been opened up. Death is a part of the life process. Individuals have thoughts and attitudes about their deaths, often influenced by their religious preference and cultural background. To allow fulfillment and continued growth of the individual, nursing must consider death as well as life.

Interventions that do not consider a person's location in time will fail; e.g., teaching aids designed for someone with a high school education will probably bore a listener who has a doctoral degree.

Stereotypes tend to inhibit the nurse's ability to approach clients as holistic individuals. Trite phrases and jokes demonstrate uncomfortableness and increase distance between the client and nurse. The nurse who is learning about the client as a total person allows the client to share in the process of exposing himself. The nurse moves within his pace following his lead.

Since each person lives in a social environment, he or she will be influenced by the events in his or her world. Political actions, financial changes, and labor strikes all affect his or her life situation. For example, opportunities for women in the 1970s differ vastly from those in the 1950s. Women in the 1970s will have different expectations and needs. There are women becoming merchant mariners, telephone installers, truck drivers, and executives.

People are able to express their sexual preferences, choose to live as married, or get married in the traditional manner. Children are no longer a given. Women have a choice about when and how many children they will have.

Nurses must remember to take into account the variances in the world today. Since nurses make up a large portion of health professionals, they are essential for changing the health-care system. Not to aid the change would be clinging to an outworn system. Since change occurs anyway, nurses may as well emphasize its constructive aspects.

---

[11] Rogers, Martha E., *An Introduction to the Theoretical Basis of Nursing*, 1970.

10 NURSING ASSESSMENT

Nurses are frequently involved in life-and-death situations. In such instances the priority for intervention is to remove any threats to life. The holistic approach to clients demands attention to maintenance of human integrity. Bower describes the criteria for priority setting as (1) threats to life, dignity, and integrity, (2) threats of destructive change, and (3) threats to normal growth and development of the individual, family, or community.[12]

The complexity of humans and their world necessitates a total assessment. The adequate health assessment must include a nursing history, which will help the nurse understand the client's place in time. It must also cover, among others, psychosocial, physical, spiritual, family, employment, and cultural aspects. Understanding a person's many aspects as he or she moves through life is a refined but essential part of adequate nursing. Nursing interventions based on a multidimensional assessment will more likely meet the total needs of clients, thus maintaining and nurturing their integrity, growth, and development.

PROGRESS CHECK

1. Which of the following areas are important for nurses to assess with their clients? Circle the correct answer(s).
   a. home environment
   b. employment situation
   c. date of birth
   d. physical complaints

Complete the following:

2. Holism is _____

3. Human beings have been described as having physical and mental aspects. There is a triad description that includes physical, mental, and _____ aspects.

4. _____ describes the continual interaction between humans and their world.

5. _____ is as much a part of life as living.

6. _____ inhibit the nurse's ability to approach clients as holistic individuals.

7. Number the items below in order of highest to lowest priority.
   a. ____ threat of destructive change to an individual, family, or community
   b. ____ threat to normal growth and development of an individual, family, or community
   c. ____ threat to life and dignity of an individual, family, or community

8. Explain the reasons for a multidimensional approach to the nursing assessment process.

ANSWERS
1. circle all
2. the approach to a human as a unified total, more than the sum of his or her parts

---

[12] Bower, Fay Louise, *The Process of Planning Nursing Care: A Practice Model*, 1976.

© 1977 Wiley

INTRODUCTION TO NURSING ASSSESSMENT **11**

3. social
4. The term homeodynamics
5. Death
6. Stereotypes
7. a. 2   b. 3   c. 1
8. A human is a complex being who cannot be understood only by studying his or her parts. A person's place in time affects his or her total being, as a person is an open system continually interacting with his or her environment.

ACTIVITY 3
MAKING AN ASSESSMENT

There are four steps in the process of making an assessment: (1) select the area(s) to be assessed, (2) gather data, (3) sort and categorize the data, and (4) write a summary statement. Each step will be discussed and demonstrated.

STEP 1: SELECT THE AREA(S) TO BE ASSESSED
An assessment can be made of any object, condition, or process. One should be clear at the outset about what is to be assessed; otherwise the assessment may be invalid or useless.

EXAMPLE 1
Mrs. Johnson, a new nursing student on a surgical ward, was told to make an assessment of a newly admitted client named Miss Tomkins, whose diagnosis was pre-op for Dilatation and Curettage (D & C). When Mrs. Johnson reached the room, she did which of the following?

1. She asked for Miss Tomkins. She then sat in the chair next to the client, introduced herself, and began to ask her questions about her previous hospitalizations.
2. She asked for Miss Tomkins, then went to the bedside, introduced herself, and began to ask questions about how she was feeling.
3. She asked for Miss Tomkins, then went to the bedside and introduced herself. She placed a thermometer in the client's mouth and began to count her pulse and respirations.
4. She asked for Miss Tomkins, then went to the bedside and introduced herself. She sat down and asked Miss Tomkins about the amount of vaginal bleeding she was having.

STEP 2: GATHER DATA
There are several ways to gather data:

Observation: Although usually thought of as visual perception, an observation may be something seen, smelled, heard, touched, or tasted. It can be the result of an experiment, a measurement, or a behavior. It is a description of examination findings.

Interview: An interview is a conversation for the purpose of gathering data. The interviewer directs the session to assure he gets the information he needs. It may be between two people or more, face-to-face, or by telephone.

Records: Records refer to clinical records and documents—an old or new chart, a birth, marriage, or death certificate, and even school records. Records contain data about past events.

Literature: Literature includes all published materials, such as books, journals, newspapers, and testing tools.

© 1977 Wiley

12 NURSING ASSESSMENT

Having selected the area(s) of assessment, one must choose one or more methods for data collection. In Example 1 Mrs. Johnson used the observation (3) and interview (1, 2, 4) methods.

Here is another example:

EXAMPLE 2
Mrs. Ina Roxe is 66 years old. She has been hospitalized on a medical ward for evaluation following a stroke in her home the previous evening. Mr. James Webb, student nurse, has been assigned to give morning nursing care to Mrs. Roxe.

1. He begins his assessment by:
   Circle the appropriate actions.
   a. choosing to assess the level of disability resulting from the stroke
   b. choosing to assess the events leading up to the stroke
   c. choosing to assess the client's home situation
   d. choosing to assess the client's present state of being
2. He continues his assessment by:
   Circle the appropriate actions.
   a. reading the clinical chart
   b. asking the team leader about the night nurse's report of the client's condition
   c. inquiring if family members have been spoken to
   d. going to the client's room

Selecting a Method of Data Collection
When one is faced with the need to make an assessment, either one is aware of the criteria for adequate assessment or one is not. Figure 1 demonstrates these positions. The criteria for assessment give direction for the method of collection necessary. Knowledge of the present is best obtained through interview and observation. Knowledge of the past is found in records. Reading the literature aids in generalizing, forming hypotheses, and making associations between past and present data.

When the Criteria for Assessment Are Known
When the criteria for assessment are known, selecting the appropriate method of data collection is relatively simple. One needs to select the method that will give the required information. For example, Mrs. Johnson is told to assess Miss Tomkins' vital signs. She knows that the criteria for assessing vital signs require measurement of blood pressure, temperature, pulse, and respiration. She then collects the equipment, goes to the client, and gathers her data. She uses the observation method of data collection.

EXAMPLE 3
Mrs. Johnson knows that the criteria for assessing bleeding include indication of the amount of blood loss, the rate of blood loss, the color and consistency of blood, and the site of blood flow. If she were told to assess the amount of vaginal bleeding, which of the following would she do? Circle the correct answer(s).

a. ask client how much bleeding has occurred
b. count discarded perineal pads
c. observe perineal pad worn by client
d. read chart

EXAMPLE 4
The criteria for assessing whether a person is oriented are: can the client identify the present time, place, space, and circumstances? Which of the following methods of data gathering would you choose? Circle the correct answer(s).

© 1977 Wiley

a. read chart
b. interview client
c. read literature
d. observe client's behavior

EXAMPLE 5

The criteria for a registered nurse are:

1. completion of an accredited school of nursing
2. successfully passing the licensing examination in the state of application, thus receiving a license to practice as a registered nurse
3. reciprocal granting of license to practice as a registered nurse in the state of application based on satisfactorily completing above in another state
4. payment of fee(s) as indicated

Mr. Ray is the Assistant Chief of Nursing at a Veterans' Administration hospital. He is interviewing a prospective employee who says she is a registered nurse. He knows that to work in a government hospital one need only be licensed in some state in the United States. The applicant states she lost her old license from her home state. Which of the following should she do to gather data for obtaining a license in the current state? Circle the correct answer(s).

a. write to school of graduation requesting transcript be sent to the licensing board of present state
b. obtain and fill out an application for licensure as a registered nurse in present state
c. request to take registered nurse examination in home state
d. pay fee as indicated on the application

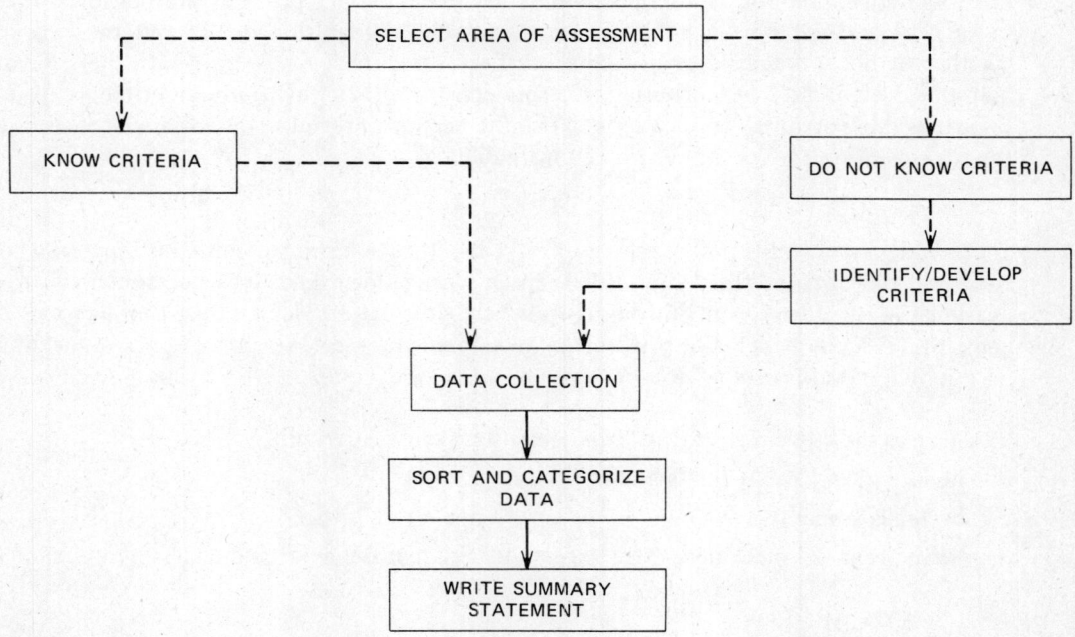

FIGURE 1
The process of making an assessment.

14 NURSING ASSESSMENT

EXAMPLE 6

The Apgar score is a method used to assess a newborn one minute after birth. The areas of assessment include heart rate, respiratory effort, muscle tone, reflex irritability, and color. Match each of the following with the appropriate method of gathering data.

____1. respiratory effort   a. record
____2. muscle tone   b. interview
____3. reflex irritability   c. observe
____4. heart rate   d. literature
____5. color

EXAMPLE 7

Mrs. Jennings appears at the emergency room where you work. She is crying and carrying a child in her arms. The child's eyes are closed and his breathing is shallow. The ABC's of trauma intervention are A–check that airway is clear, B–check for breathing, and C–check for circulation. The nurse needs data in this situation. Which method(s) should be used first? Circle the correct answer(s).

1. interview the child
2. request previous records of child's presence at the hospital
3. take the child's vital signs
4. interview the child's mother
5. read article on childhood accidents

When the Criteria for Assessment Are Unknown

Reading literature is one way of obtaining assessment criteria when they are unknown. If one wanted to know how to assess a child's level of functioning, she could go to the literature and find out about the numerous developmental scales. They would provide information about types of tasks a child should be capable of at various chronological ages. The literature would reveal whether or not a standard or criterion has been developed. Knowing what others have done can help one design one's own criteria for assessment. Another way to obtain criteria is to interview a knowledgable person. A third way is to use the person's previous state as a source of criteria; here the records of past observations prove invaluable.

EXAMPLE 8

John Addeny began his first teaching job last month. He has a student, Jim Langer, who has been sitting in the back of the room. Jim keeps his head down and does not contribute to class discussions. Mr. Addeny wants to discuss this behavior, but Jim leaves the room as soon as the class ends. Mr. Addeny believes he must make an assessment—status report—to the student's advisor.
    Which of the following does he do?

a. he uses the student's previous behaviors in his class as criteria
b. he interviews the student's advisor
c. he reads student's file
d. he reads an article called "Motivation and Student Behavior and Classroom Climate"

EXAMPLE 9

Judy Baum has never assessed a person's communication pattern before. She doesn't know any criteria for making this type of assessment. She does which of the following? Circle the correct answer(s).

© 1977 Wiley

a. reads the book, *Modern Technology to Aid Communication Systems*
b. has a conversation with a client and tape records interview
c. reads three articles on styles of communication
d. interviews a psychologist on commonly encountered communication patterns

STEP 3: SORT AND CATEGORIZE THE DATA

Once you have collected the data, they need to be sorted and categorized for use. Usually data are gathered from a number of sources and in a variety of ways. When data are sorted and categorized, relationships begin to emerge. Remember Miss Tomkins in Example 1; data could have been gathered about several areas. Since Mrs. Johnson didn't know which area to assess, she spent about a half hour interviewing the client. She learned the following:

Miss Tomkins is 30 years old and newly married. She does not use her married name because of her business. This is her and her husband's first attempt at having a baby. She aborted the fetus two weeks ago. She has been bleeding continually since. Miss Tomkins tells Mrs. Johnson that she really wants a baby and fears she may never be able to have one. She further says she is nervous about being in the hospital: "Everything's so strange." Mrs. Johnson takes her temperature, pulse, respiration, and blood pressure. The readings are: temperature 101° rectally; pulse 96; respiration 20; and blood pressure 98/50. There are five used perineal pads in the bag at the bedside. The present pad, Miss Tomkins says, has been on for about one hour. It is saturated with bright red blood, no clots. Mrs. Johnson returns to the nurses' station and begins to sort these data. She sets up some categories as shown below.

Present Condition	*Health History*	*Family History*
Vaginal bleeding at rate of one perineal pad per hour. Blood pressure 90/50; temperature 101° rectally; pulse 96; respiration 20	Aborted two weeks ago and bleeding continually since	No data

Financial Status	*Spirituality*	*Feelings*
Businesswoman	No data	Fearful may not be able to have a child. Wants very much to have a child

Significant Others

Married—husband

Mrs. Johnson can immediately see areas in which she needs additional data. She reports vital-sign data to the charge nurse and begins to read the client's chart. A nursing history, physical examination, and social history have been completed. She obtains the following data:

According to the chart, Miss Tomkins' last blood pressure—four hours ago—was 110/60, pulse 90, and respiration 20. Her temperature was 99° rectally. The last peripad count was four hours ago.

Miss Tomkins is the oldest of three children. She has two younger sisters. Her parents reside in another state. Her sisters live with their parents. She moved to this state to start a business called Hostesses, Ltd., with a girlfriend. The girlfriend sold her part of the business to Miss Tomkins two months after they opened. She married her husband, Gene Saunders, shortly thereafter. They have been married two years. They decided six months ago to attempt to have a

© 1977 Wiley

16 NURSING ASSESSMENT

baby. She had been on birth control pills for about five years prior. Stated she has always been healthy. She belongs to a health spa, has had no previous hospitalizations, has attended outpatient clinics, and has health insurance. Her husband, a college instructor, is currently unemployed. She is scheduled for surgery at 8 o'clock this evening.

Sort the above data into appropriate categories.

Present Condition

Four hours ago: temperature rectally 99°; blood pressure 110/60; pulse 90; and respiration 20
Last perineal pad count was four hours ago
Surgery scheduled for 8 o'clock this evening

Health History

Says always been healthy
No previous hospitalizations
Belongs to a health spa
Had been on birth control pills for five years

Family History

Parents reside in another state with two sisters
Married two years
Decided to have baby six months ago

Financial Status

Started own business with girlfriend; now sole owner
Has health insurance
Husband is unemployed; a college instructor

Spirituality

No data

Feelings

No additional data

Significant Others

Husband's name is Gene Saunders
Has two younger sisters, live in another state
Parents live in another state

Do you see any other areas in which data are needed in order to make an adequate assessment? Perhaps you said psychological, spiritual, educational, home environment, work environment, hobbies, and interests. There are more. You are on the right track if you stated any of the above.

EXAMPLE 10

Sort and categorize the following data:

Andrea Brown is a four-year-old black girl who has been brought to the clinic for a hearing evaluation. Her mother says the kindergarten teacher requested it because Andrea doesn't pay attention to classroom activities. Andrea smiles at you and you smile back. You start to ask her questions. You ask her name and age. She answers all your questions. She looks into your eyes throughout the conversation. Since she is early for her appointment, you ask her if she would like to play in the toy room while waiting. She says yes, and follows you. Once in the room she immediately goes to the window ledge and climbs up looking outside. You ask her what she is looking at and she says, "I am looking for a squirrel." Upon further discussion you find that there is a squirrel she calls "Fuzzy" who lives in a tree near school. She watches him every day and feeds him at recess and after school. She says she is worried because she hasn't seen him in three days. She says she hopes he didn't die but if he did, "I know he's in heaven with God." She says he's her only friend and starts to cry.

© 1977 Wiley

STEP 4: WRITE AN ASSESSMENT STATEMENT

The last step in making an assessment is to write a summary statement of your data collection. The assessment summary does not include value judgments or recommendations; it is a statement of what exists. It should be limited to between three and five sentences. The reader of the assessment statement can then proceed to develop his own interpretations, identify problems, and begin to generate alternative interventions.

Review Example 8, Mr. Addeny and Jim Langer. A summary statement would be:

"Jim Langer, a nursing student, formerly contributed to class. After the first exam, his participation stopped. He received a grade of 80. His records show him to be a high achiever who believes an 80 is unsatisfactory."

Answers

Example 1: Item 4 was the intervention with the highest priority, as bleeding is considered life threatening. Following 4, all of the others were correct. Mrs. Johnson was not told specifically which area to assess. An adequate initial assessment of this client's condition would include all of these. Although Mrs. Johnson knew the client was newly admitted, she did not know whether an initial assessment had been made.

Example 2: 1. Mr. Webb may choose to begin with any of these areas. However, a and d are more relevant to the present situation. Since he has been assigned Mrs. Roxe's immediate nursing care, these two areas have priority over b and c.
2. If Mr. Webb is to assess Mrs. Roxe's level of disability from the stroke and her present state of being, a, b, and d are appropriate interventions. Nursing intervention a is an example of gathering data from a record. Intervention b is an example of interviewing. The intervention for c is an observation example.

Example 3: The correct answers are a, b, c, and d. The first three give information about the present state of vaginal bleeding. Reading the chart provides information about the past that needs to be considered in assessing the client's present condition. The methods to gather data are interviewing, observation, and records.

© 1977 Wiley

Example 4: The correct answers are a and b. Answer a can give you information about the last person's assessment. The client may demonstrate the same or a differing level of orientation, which then becomes a part of the assessment. An interview of the client asking him if he knows where he is, the date, and how he came to be where he is can give data for assessment of orientation at that moment. The methods used to gather data here were records and interview. One did not need to go the literature, since the criteria were known. Observing behavior may or may not have given accurate data for orientation, a cognitive function.

Example 5: Answers a, b, and d are correct. In addition, she may need to write a letter to the licensing board of her home state authorizing them to release information about her performance on the licensing examination. Answer c is incorrect. She could write to her home state requesting a new copy of her license, but she need not rewrite the exam. Should she not be granted a reciprocal license, she would need to take the licensing exam in the present state.

Example 6: The correct answer for each one is c. Remember: observation includes the use of all five senses. It also includes a measurement. The heart rate is obtained by using a stethoscope. Respiratory effort is assessed by observing the chest rising and falling and listening for the quality of the cry. Muscle tone and reflex irritability require looking and touching. A determination of color requires vision.

Example 7: The appropriate methods of data collection are numbers 3 and 5. Immediately the child's physical state needs assessing. Next the mother is interviewed to obtain data about what happened.

Example 8: All the responses are correct. Mr. Addeny recalls that Jim often raised his hand to make contributions in the class until a month ago. He also notes that the first exam occurred a month ago. His record book shows that Jim received an 80 on the exam. Jim's student file shows that he usually gets grades in the 90s. Interviewing Jim's advisor, Mr. Addeny learns that Jim has a strong desire to be a nurse. Achievement of good grades is very important to Jim; he doesn't consider an 80 satisfactory. The article describes how a motivated student can be turned off by certain classroom environments and how the turned-off student behaves. Mr. Addeny can begin to develop his own criteria for assessing when a student is becoming discouraged.

Example 9: Only c and d are correct. Articles on communication styles would help her begin developing some criteria to make assessments of her client's communication patterns. A psychologist is an appropriate resource person for criteria. Answer b is inappropriate because she doesn't know the criteria for assessment yet. Answer a has nothing to do with assessing individual communication styles.

When developing criteria for assessment, read for statements about what most people experience, do, or say. Look for common ideas that recur from one reading to another. Then list common patterns and characteristics for future reference. It is like developing your own special recipe. You go to several cookbooks to get an idea of what should be there; then through your own experiences you modify the recipe accordingly.

Example 10: Below is a list of possible categories:

Home Environment	Interests/Hobbies	Motor Behavior
School Environment	Present Condition	Health History
Spirituality	Psychosocial Condition	Education

A possible sorting of the data under these categories might look like this:

Home Environment	*School Environment*	*Interests/Hobbies*
No data given	Teacher says she doesn't pay attention	Watching and feeding squirrels

© 1977 Wiley

Spirituality

Believes in God
Believes in heaven

Present Condition

Answered all nurses's questions
At clinic for hearing test

Psychosocial Condition

Worried about her squirrel
Smiles when smiled at
Has eye contact
No friends

Health History

No data given

Motor Behavior

Climbed up onto window ledge

Education

In kindergarten

How many categories did you have? Select areas that will help you understand the total person.

PROGRESS CHECK

Review Example 1, Miss Tomkins. Write a summary statement below.

ANSWER

Miss Tomkins, a 30-year-old woman, aborted two weeks ago and has been bleeding continuously since then. She is hospitalized for a Dilatation and Curettage. This is her and her husband's first attempt at having children. She is fearful that she will not bear children. She has shown a drop in blood pressure to 98/50 and an elevated temperature at 101° rectally.

SUMMARY

The assessment process described can be used to assess any item, process, or condition. It can be used to assess a group such as a family as well as to assess a community. The steps are (1) select area of assessment, (2) gather data, (3) sort and categorize data, and (4) write assessment summary statement.

For an additional activity, select a family or community for assessment. Then proceed through the process. What do you want to assess about the family: communication styles, support systems, or coalitions? What about the community? Transportation adequacy, location of and number of schools, stores, police, fire department, etc.? There are multiple resources for data if criteria are unknown. Once you learn the steps, you will find yourself using the process repeatedly.

© 1977 Wiley

20 NURSING ASSESSMENT

POSTTEST

1. Match the following words with the correct definition.
   - ____ a. interpretive statement made at the completion of the assessment judgment
   - ____ b. comparison of data for deciding worth
   - ____ c. gathering data, sorting and categorizing, and summary statement
   - ____ d. explanation of the meaning of data
   - ____ e. comparing data and forming an opinion about data's relationship

   1. evaluation
   2. judgment
   3. diagnosis
   4. interpretation
   5. assessment

2. The steps in the process of making an assessment are:
   Select the letter with the correct combination.
   a. review literature, write criteria of assessment, sort and categorize data, and apply to situation.
   b. select area to assess, gather data, sort and categorize data, and write assessment statement.
   c. evaluate needs of individual, sort and categorize needs, select an area of need, and write an intervention.
   d. list the criteria for assessment, interview the client, sort and categorize data, and write interview summary.

3. Match the situation with the method of data collection used.
   - ____ 1. reading a book on the communication process
   - ____ 2. speaking to a mother about her child's condition
   - ____ 3. spending the day with the team leader to learn what her job entails
   - ____ 4. reading a client's chart

   a. interview
   b. records
   c. observation
   d. literature

4. Describe the following as methods of data collection:
   a. interview

   b. records

   c. observation

   d. literature

5. The criteria for providing nursing care include making a nursing care plan based on client's needs, developing and implementing nursing interventions, and then evaluating intervention.

© 1977 Wiley

Which of the following would be sources of data about the above? Circle the correct answer(s).
   a. records
   b. interview
   c. literature
   d. observation

6. The criteria for isolation of a person with hepatitis are unknown to the nurse. She has a client just admitted with the diagnosis. Which of the following can she do?
   a. call the engineer
   b. call the infection control nurse
   c. request a book from the library on isolation techniques
   d. place the client in a semiprivate room until she learns criteria

7. Read the following situation. Sort and categorize the data. Identify at least five categories.
     Janet is a 16-year-old Chicana. She attends high school and was receiving excellent grades until this year. During the summer she gained a lot of weight. A visit to the physician finally uncovered a hormone imbalance. Although she is taking medication and sticking to her diet, she is much heavier than before. A former student leader, she now stays to herself. She no longer goes out on weekend nights. She describes herself as ugly and lonely. Her grades are falling. You are the school nurse. She tells you, "What's the use, I may as well eat what I want." She had an argument with her best girlfriend. Her parents are supportive. Her two younger brothers and sister tease her about her weight.

8. Write an assessment statement for the situation in Question 7.

9. Write a definition of the term holism.

© 1977 Wiley

22 NURSING ASSESSMENT

10. Explain the phrase "a multidimensional nursing assessment."

11. The first priority of the threats to man's safety is the threat to _____.

12. The (a) threat to normal growth and development and the (b) threat to destructive change are two other threats to man, the family, and community. Which comes next (after the answer to 11) in order of priority, a or b? ____.

Answers

1. a. 3   b. 1   c. 5   d. 4   e. 2
2. b
3. 1. d   2. a   3. c or a   4. b
4. a. interview: a directed conversation for purpose of obtaining data. It may be between two or more people
   b. records: documents; descriptions of past events
   c. observation: a measurement or result of an experiment; the results of use of five senses for examination
   d. literature: all published materials
5. all of them
6. b or c

7.
Present Condition	*Education*	*Social Condition*
Overweight	Attends high school	No dates on weekends
Threatening to go off diet	Was getting good grades; now grades are falling	Recent argument with best friend
Still has hormone imbalance		Sixteen years old
		Staying to self
		Former student leader
		Lonely

Family	*Health History*	*Self-Esteem*
Lives with parents, two brothers and sister	Development of hormone imbalance last year	Sees self as ugly
All siblings younger than her	Managed by medication and diet	*Culture*
Siblings tease her about weight gain		Chicana
Parents are supportive		

8. Janet, a 16-year-old Chicana, developed a hormone imbalance, which created an overweight condition. Condition is managed by diet and medication. She has been withdrawing and her school grades are suffering. Parents are supportive, but siblings tease her. She sees herself as ugly.

9. Holism is a concept used to depict man as a unified whole. It emphasizes his integrity and interaction with his environment.

© 1977 Wiley

10. A multidimensional nursing assessment acknowledges the holistic view of man. It attempts to achieve that goal by assessing the total client rather than a part. The dimensions and their interrelations help one to see the total individual.
11. life
12. b

References

Bloch, Doris, "Some Crucial Terms in Nursing—What Do They Really Mean?" *Nursing Outlook* 22 (1974): 689–694.

Bower, Fay Louise, *The Process of Planning Nursing Care: A Practice Model.* St. Louis: The C. V. Mosby Co., 1976, pp. 14, 45.

Doona, Mary Ellen, "The Judgment Process in Nursing," *Image* 8 (1976): 27–29.

Lewis, Lucille, *Planning Patient Care.* Dubuque, Iowa: Wm. C. Brown Co., 1970, p. 77.

Rogers, Martha E., *An Introduction to the Theoretical Basis of Nursing.* Philadelphia: F. A. Davis Co., 1970.

Webster's New World Dictionary. New York: The World Publishing Co., 1964, pp. 88, 792, 502, 764, 403.

Wolanin, Mary Opal, "Nursing Assessment," *Nursing and the Aged,* edited by Irene M. Burnside. New York: McGraw-Hill Book Co., 1976.

TONI HEILMAN, R.N., M.S.

WILEY NURSING CONCEPT MODULE

THE NURSING HISTORY

CONTENTS
PRETEST 27   Answers 30
INTRODUCTION 31
TERMINAL OBJECTIVES 32
    ACTIVITY 1. The Client History Process 32
    ACTIVITY 2. The Client History Content: Physical-Cultural Human Needs 34
    ACTIVITY 3. The Client History Content: Psycho-Sociocultural Human Needs 40
    ACTIVITY 4. The Client History Content: Coping Mechanisms 45
    ACTIVITY 5. The Client History Content: Alternatives in Input 47
POSTTEST 51   Answers 55
REFERENCES 55

PRETEST

1. A client history is:
   a. the same as a medical history
   b. the same as a nursing history
   c. a process of gathering facts about client problems
   d. a method of ascertaining client coping behaviors
      1. b and c
      2. b, c, and d
      3. all of the above
      4. none of the above

2. A client history:
   a. obtains a data base for determining nursing actions
   b. reviews signs and symptoms in order to make a medical diagnosis
   c. makes inferences about nursing actions that are called for
   d. identifies a client's usual pattern of coping with stress
      1. c only
      2. a and d
      3. all of the above
      4. none of the above

3. Internal environment in the interviewer includes:
   a. eye contact
   b. knowledge of the questionnaire content
   c. absence of noise
   d. freedom from pain
      1. b only
      2. b and c
      3. c and d
      4. all of the above

4. You can establish a climate of trust in the client by:
   a. talking about the weather
   b. saying, "I trust you, therefore you should trust me"
   c. beginning the interview with nonthreatening questions
   d. giving the client your undivided attention
      1. a and b
      2. a and c
      3. b and d
      4. c and d

5. Which of the following statements are true?
   a. A client history is not necessary for a patient who is being hospitalized overnight.
   b. Only one format is acceptable for obtaining a client history.
   c. Begin the history with nonintrusive questions; then proceed to more sensitive areas.
   d. The best source of information is the client himself.
      1. a and b
      2. a and c
      3. b and c
      4. c and d

6. Identify the basic needs of man.
   a. respiration, nutrition, elimination
   b. affiliation, achievement

© 1977 Wiley

27

28 NURSING ASSESSMENT

      c. safety
      d. sexuality
         1. a only
         2. a and c
         3. all of the above
         4. none of the above

7. Identify "alterations in input," as distinct from basic needs:
    a. pain
    b. sexuality
    c. anxiety
    d. sensory deprivation
       1. d only
       2. a and d
       3. b and c
       4. a, c, and d

8. Which of the following statements is/are true?
    a. Seventy-five percent of all communication is nonverbal.
    b. The client is always a reliable source of information.
    c. The client history is the same as a medical history.
    d. Anyone, with training, can take a client history.
       1. a only
       2. a and b
       3. b and c
       4. b, c, and d

9. The essential elements of a client history are:
    a. record of name, age, sex, vital signs, height and weight
    b. assessment of basic needs
    c. determination of alterations in input
    d. adaptation of questions to age and sex
       1. a, b, and d
       2. b, c, and d
       3. all of the above
       4. none of the above

10. Formats that are acceptable for use in obtaining a client history are:
    a. question and answer
    b. narrative
    c. nursing-care plan
    d. medical history
       1. a and b
       2. a and c
       3. b and d
       4. c and d

Situation: Jimmy Brown is a fifteen-year-old who has been admitted to Pediatrics with suspected juvenile-onset diabetes. The following four questions relate to Jimmy.

11. A client history will:
    a. determine Jimmy's usual activities of daily living
    b. prove that Jimmy has diabetes
    c. state several plans for teaching Jimmy about diabetes
    d. identify Jimmy's pattern of behavior for coping with stress
       1. a and d
       2. a and b

© 1977 Wiley

3. c and d
4. b and d

12. A good way to begin to establish a trust relationship with Jimmy would be to:
    a. Talk about his hobbies
    b. Ask him how he feels about hospitalization
    c. Say, "There are lots of other boys your age who have diabetes"
    d. Tell him how important it is for you to get this history
    1. a only
    2. b only
    3. b and c
    4. a, c, and d

13. Of the following, which are Jimmy's basic needs?
    a. to feel part of a group
    b. dietary restrictions
    c. knowledge of basic hygiene
    d. identification with masculinity
    1. a and b
    2. a and d
    3. b, c, and d
    4. all of the above

14. Jimmy has been reported to be very hostile (verbally and physically abusive) today—the time of admission. Which of the following actions is recommended?
    a. Assign the nursing history to a nurse's aide whom Jimmy appears to trust.
    b. Make up a nursing history with information obtained from the medical history.
    c. Forego the client history.
    d. Interview Jimmy's parents with the intent to complete the form at a time when Jimmy is agreeable.

Situation: Mrs. Lewis is a 35-year-old woman who has just been admitted for a radical mastectomy. The doctor tells you the client is very upset because her husband is leaving her because she will "no longer be a woman." The following four questions relate to Mrs. Lewis.

15. You enter Mrs. Lewis' room to take a client history and find her lying in bed weeping. What is your *best* first action?
    a. Get her some medication for pain.
    b. Ask her, "Would you like to share your problem with me?"
    c. Ignore her weeping and begin the history.
    d. Tell her, "There's no use in crying—it won't solve your problem."
    1. a only
    2. b only
    3. a and c
    4. a and d

16. A comprehensive client history will:
    a. Describe Mrs. Lewis' depression.
    b. Identify Mrs. Lewis' concept of sexuality.
    c. State Mrs. Lewis' usual coping behaviors.
    d. Identify the relationship that exists between Mr. and Mrs. Lewis.
    1. b and d
    2. a, c, and d
    3. all of the above
    4. none of the above

17. Which are desirable actions for the nurse who interviews Mrs. Lewis for the first time?
    a. Listen for cues to Mrs. Lewis' self-concept.

© 1977 Wiley

30 NURSING ASSESSMENT

    b. Persist with questions that will fully reveal Mrs. Lewis' sexuality problems.
    c. Relate Mrs. Lewis' crying to fear, anxiety, and depression.
    d. Understand nonverbal cues that may reveal Mrs. Lewis' feelings about sexuality.
       1. a and c
       2. b and d
       3. a, c, and d
       4. all of the above

18. Part of Mrs. Lewis' "internal environment" may include:
    a. knitting while being interviewed
    b. freedom from pain
    c. having privacy during the interview
    d. being "at ease" with the interviewer
       1. a and b
       2. a and d
       3. b and c
       4. b and d

19. Listed below are six categories you might use when taking a client history. For each category, state one question that would be specific for obtaining information about a twelve-month-old child.
    a. rest:

    b. diet:

    c. safety:

    d. communication:

    e. activity:

    f. coping behavior:

Answers

1. 2	7. 4	13. 4
2. 3	8. 1	14. d
3. 3	9. 3	15. 2
4. 4	10. 1	16. 3
5. 4	11. 1	17. 3
6. 3	12. 1	18. 3

Examples of correct responses may include questions concerning:

    a. rest: nap times, hours of sleep at any given rest period, sound or light sleeper
    b. diet: formula (amounts), food, digestive difficulties, allergies, regurgitation

© 1977 Wiley

c. safety: crib, surroundings (cupboards, medicine chests, cleaning agents, wall plugs, paint and plaster, appliances, garbage disposal), babysitter, clothing
d. communication: words or sounds that have special meaning, connotation; hugging, rocking behaviors
e. activity: toys related to age, indoor/outdoor activities, crawling and walking attempts
f. coping: manifestations of anxiety (anger, unusual crying, withdrawal, unusual quiet, vomiting, fear)

INTRODUCTION

Nurses have been making assessments of patients, or clients, since nursing began. One extremely valuable part of the assessment is taking the client history. Since nursing has become more complex in theory and practice, it has become necessary to develop more sophisticated tools for gaining pertinent information from clients. This module provides a method of client interview that will obtain a comprehensive, accurate, and useful data base from which to identify client problems and plan effective care.

Taking a client history is the process by which a nurse ascertains facts about the client's basic needs, problems, and coping behaviors. The client is any man, woman, child, social group, or family unit. The client may be well or ill, or at any point along the wellness-illness continuum, and in need of nursing intervention. The initial interview is usually part of the *assessment* step of the *nursing process*.

The nurse's interview of the client, referred to as the "client history" or "nursing history," differs from the medical history. A medical history records past and present signs and symptoms. Information is gathered in such a manner as to facilitate medical diagnosis and prescription of treatment. A nursing history, or client history, reviews the client's systems in order to obtain information about his basic needs and coping behaviors. Specific nursing needs are identified so that interventions can be individualized. These interventions will incorporate the client's functional coping behaviors. With the emphasis now on participatory care by the client, it is more important than ever for the client and the nurse to develop a mutual base of information.

The best source of information for a client history is the client. But sometimes the client is unable to give the information—for example, in cases of severe injury accompanied by temporary loss of memory, confusion, or unconsciousness. In such cases the history must be gained from a significant other, such as spouse, relative, or friend. In the case of infants and toddlers the parents are usually the most reliable source of information.

Certain interviewer qualities are necessary for the acquisition of a complete nursing history. The interviewer needs well-developed communication skills and the ability to ask questions in such a way as to obtain the information sought. She needs knowledge of the client's bio-psycho-sociocultural composition to assure comprehension of the totality of the information. Therefore, by virtue of their educational backgrounds, students of nursing and registered nurses are the persons best qualified to take a client history.

Prerequisites to this Module

1. A course in "Communications" or "Communication Skills."
2. Listen to tapes 3, 4, 5, 6, 7, 8, 9, 11 and 14 from *Nursing Communication Skills*.[1]

---

[1] Roe, Anne K.; Sherwood, Mary C.; and Dunham, Frances, *Nursing Communication Skills*, 1975.

© 1977 Wiley

Instructions to the Learner

This module is set up to facilitate your learning how to take a client history. You are expected to follow the steps sequentially, first learning the basic components in the history-taking process, then moving into the more complex areas of coping mechanisms and illness.

Taking a nursing history is perfected only with much practice. It is therefore suggested that you "practice" many times with friends and relatives. In this way you will gain mastery in the process before you ever approach your first client.

Do not be discouraged if you come out of an interview and realize you've forgotten a whole section of questions. Simply return to the client (if feasible) and fill in the blanks. The client will probably be much more understanding than you expected.

STEPS

1. Complete the prerequisite work.
2. Take the Pretest. Grade yourself.
3. Study the content through to Activity 2.
4. Complete the Progress Check following Activity 2.
5. Study the content of Activities 3, 4, and 5 and complete the Progress Check at the end of each Activity.
6. Practice taking a history on five "well" persons.
7. Practice taking a history on five persons who are experiencing alterations in input.
8. Take the Posttest. You should score better than you did on the Pretest.

TERMINAL OBJECTIVES

Upon completion of this module the student will be able to:

1. define "client history"
2. state four rationales for taking a client history
3. identify external and internal environments requisite for an optimum client history
4. prepare an outline that includes the basic needs of man and alterations in input
5. demonstrate, in writing, two methods of recording a client history
6. relate the basic history of a given client to his alternatives in input
7. adapt the nursing history format for use with a child

ACTIVITY 1

THE CLIENT HISTORY PROCESS

A course in communication skills is a prerequisite of this module. Therefore, this part will emphasize those skills especially desirable for taking a comprehensive, informative nursing history.

© 1977 Wiley

Environment

The environment in which a nursing history is taken includes both the exterior and interior milieu. External environmental features include privacy, neutral surroundings, and absence of distracting noises. An office or a private room is an appropriate external setting. The interviewer should be seated, at about eye level with the client, at a distance of about 2 to 3 feet. The client should be seated in a comfortable chair or lying in bed.

The internal environment is important for the nurse as well as for the client. The nurse needs to be relaxed and prepared (by knowing the content of the interview). Conveying self-assurance and warmth to the client is important. The client should be helped to feel relatively comfortable with the interviewer. Some of this can be accomplished by making sure that the client is relatively free from pain and understands the purpose of the interview.

TYPES OF QUESTIONS TO ASK THE CLIENT

When taking a nursing history, the interviewer needs very quickly to establish a climate of trust with someone who usually begins as a perfect stranger. Very personal and intrusive questions will be asked. Therefore, the interviewer should convey genuine interest in what the client is saying by maintaining eye contact most of the time and by giving undivided attention all of the time. The interview begins with nonthreatening, broad, general questions; questions about activity, diet, and respiration are appropriate. As trust is established, the client will be more likely to respond openly and honestly to sensitive questions.

It helps to be prepared for the interview by knowing what kinds of questions and general categories are going to be covered. Minimizing questions that can be answered by a simple "Yes" or "No" is important. Use open-ended questions that stimulate the client to expand on the responses. "How . . . ," "how much . . . ," "how often . . . ," "who . . . ," and "where . . ." questions are better than "why . . . ," "does . . . ," and "is . . ." questions.

Examples: Open-ended questions: "How do you usually exercise most of the time?" "How much water do you usually drink throughout the day and night?" "How often do you take aspirin and how many?" "Who is the most important person in your life?" "Where is the pain?"

Undesirable types of questions: "Why do you practice premarital sex?" (Judgmental)

And sometimes there are questions that will go unanswered indefinitely.

Success of the interview depends on proper external and internal environment, content of questions and responses, and cooperation of the client with the interviewer. If these requirements are fulfilled, the nursing history should contain all the information necessary to make nursing assessments and nursing plans.

An interview of a "well" person, such as a yearly physical, should take about a half hour. An interview of a person with many problems can take as much as an hour or more. If the patient is sick, it may be well to complete the interview in small time segments, in order to conserve his or her energy.

PROGRESS CHECK

Answer the following questions:

1   What is a client history?

2. How does a nursing history differ from a medical history?

3. What are four rationales for taking a client history?

© 1977 Wiley

34 NURSING ASSESSMENT

    4. What is "internal environment"?

    5. Name some "external environment" features requisite to taking a good nursing history.

ANSWERS
1. Page 31.
2. Page 31.
3. Page 31.
4. Page 33.
5. Page 33.

ACTIVITY 2
THE CLIENT HISTORY CONTENT: PHYSICAL-CULTURAL HUMAN NEEDS

There are several ways in which a nursing history may be accomplished. Some nurses prefer to give the client a small questionnaire, then go over it after he has filled it out. Other nurses prefer to complete the history solely by means of interview. Either method is acceptable if it gets the necessary information.

No matter what format is used the nurse should be well organized and comprehensive with approach. A comprehensive format is suggested below, and it is further suggested that the format be committed to memory in the order presented, so that the client history may be taken methodically.

The format begins with broad, general questions that are relatively nonthreatening, then proceeds to categories that are more intrusive into the person's innermost feelings and, therefore, more threatening. Hopefully, the client will be willing to respond to the more personal questions because he has gained a certain trust relationship with the interviewer.

Every person has certain basic needs that must be fulfilled. (See Figure 1.) Some needs are more important to some persons than others, and needs often change in priority throughout life. Alterations in input will cause priorities of needs to change. An infant needs to be fed, be dry, be kept warm, and be nurtured. The child has a need to become independent in feeding, eliminating, and in clothing itself, yet it still shares the need for nurturance with the infant. An adult needs to fulfill social needs by seeking human relationships outside the family. Adult needs change from nurturance to those of nurturing others. An aged person may retain independence or may become dependent on someone to fill basic needs, such as food, clothing, and shelter.

Examples of alterations in input are illness, anxiety, pain, poverty, loss, and death. Such alterations will have important effects on a person's basic needs, and if they are present, coping mechanisms need to be assessed. (See Figures 2 and 3.)

The following history form is intended for use when interviewing a well person. The information sought can be expected from an adult, but certain revisions will be necessary when gathering data about an infant or a child. The form is unstructured so that it may be adapted to the interviewer's particular requirements.

© 1977 Wiley

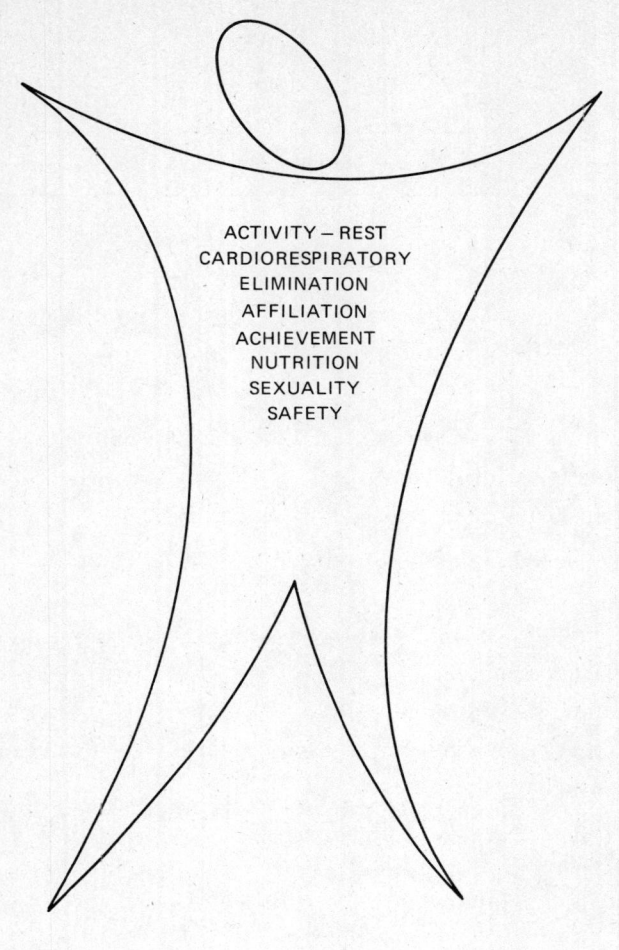

FIGURE 1
The basic needs applicable to all persons.

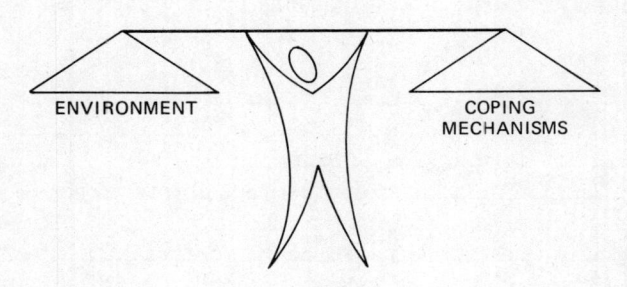

ACTIVITY – REST
CARDIORESPIRATORY
ELIMINATION
AFFILIATION
ACHIEVEMENT
NUTRITION
SEXUALITY
SAFETY

FIGURE 2
The individual in balance with the environment.

ENVIRONMENT
COPING MECHANISMS

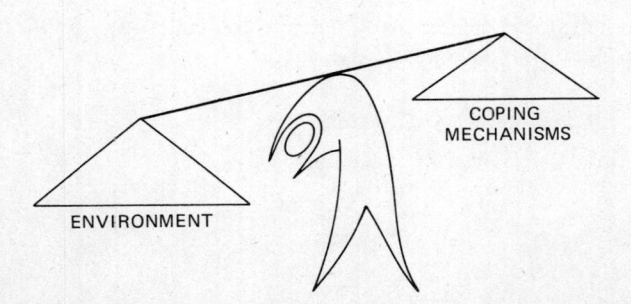

FIGURE 3
The individual in stress—unable to cope with the environment.

ENVIRONMENT
COPING MECHANISMS

© 1977 Wiley

36 NURSING ASSESSMENT

History Form

BASIC INFORMATION
Name_____ Age_____ Sex _____
Height_____ Weight_____ B.P._____ Pulse _____
Educational Accomplishments _____
Occupation _____

ACTIVITY—REST
These questions should help you assess the usual activities of daily living. They will also help you appraise the client's pattern of rest.

Sample Questions
1. I see that your occupation is _____. How long have you worked at this job?
2. How many hours a day do you usually spend at work?
3. Would you call your work vigorous, heavy, medium, light, or sedentary?
4. Tell me what you do on a typical day, hour by hour.
5. What are your hobbies?
6. How often do you engage in your hobbies? (Daily, weekly, monthly?)
7. How do you usually spend your leisure time?
8. Are these activities vigorous, medium, light, sedentary?
9. Do you exercise? Do you think you get enough exercise? What do you do when you exercise?
10. How many hours of sleep do you usually get?
11. Do you usually have to get up at night? Why?
12. Do you rest during the day? Nap? When? For how long?
13. Do you feel rested when you arise in the morning?

Supplement
These questions relate to some alteration in activity or rest that may be experienced by a healthy person:

Eye Glasses_____ Reading only_____ All the time _____
Farsighted_____ Nearsighted_____
Dentures_____ Partial_____ Complete_____ Hearing aid _____
Artificial limb(s)_____ Impaired movement (paraplegia, etc., controlled) _____
_____ Any joint pain _____
Any uncoordinated movements_____ Describe _____

CARDIORESPIRATORY
These questions are meant to assess respiratory, cardiac, and dermatological status. Some history of cardiac and pulmonary problems in the family is also elicited.

1. Do you ever have a problem with breathing? At rest? After exertion?
2. Do you have any drainage from the nose? Throat?
3. Do you have a chronic cough?
4. Do you smoke? Packs per day _____ Cigarettes per day _____ Pipe _____ Cigars _____ Marijuana _____
5. Do you have any pain when you breathe deeply? Cough?

© 1977 Wiley

6. Is there a history of respiratory disease (cancer, emphysema, T. B., COPD, asthma) in your family?
7. How many pillows do you use at night?
8. Do you get colds more than once a year? How often? What symptoms do you have? What do you do about them?
9. Do you have any allergies that affect the skin? Rash? Blotches?
10. Do you have any allergies that bring on sneezing, sinus, etc.
11. Do you have any unusual marks on your skin? Birthmarks? Any changes in the skin lately? Scars?
12. Have you noticed any change in your hair? Excessive flaking? Itching? Thinning?
13. Do you ever have chest pain? When?
14. Have you ever had problems with your circulation?
15. Have you ever had problems with blood clotting?
16. Have you ever had problems with your blood pressure?
17. Have you ever had palpitations, or a feeling that your heart is beating faster than normal?
18. Is there a history of heart disease, CVA, clotting, circulatory disease in your family? (Who? When? What happened?)

Supplement
Remember that if any of the above questions is answered in such a way that there may be evidence of a disease process in existence, further questions need to be asked in order to clarify and elaborate on the problem.
   Respiratory: Problems with breathing? When? How long does the problem last? What aggravates the problem? What makes the problem go away?
   Chest pain? Describe the pain (sharp, dull, stabbing, intermittent, continuous, burning, radiating, deep, peripheral).
   Always ask the client if he is on any regular respiratory or cardiac medication.

NUTRITION
An assessment of the client's dietary habits will help determine nutritional status. Also, correlations can be made with activity and economic status.

1. How many meals do you usually eat per day? Snacks?
2. Do you eat in a regular pattern?
3. What are the surroundings in which you eat? Noisy, calm, hurried?
4. Tell me what you eat in a typical day.
5. What are your special food likes? Dislikes? Allergies?
6. Do you have any problems with chewing? Swallowing? Belching? Nausea?
7. Do you take any food supplements such as vitamins, Geritol? What are they, and how much, how often? Any antacids?
8. How many glasses of water, juice, pop, coffee, etc. do you usually drink in a 24-hour period?
9. How much beer, wine, other liquor do you drink per day?

Supplement
Be sure to determine any subcultural dietary habits, such as "natural foods," Spanish-American foods, Italian foods, etc. Also, be careful about the wording when asking about intake of alcohol. This may be a sensitive area if the person has any guilt feelings. Be very nonjudgmental in your reaction to his response.

© 1977 Wiley

ELIMINATION

The purpose of this assessment is to gain information regarding the client's bowel and bladder habits. This may be a somewhat embarrassing area. This category of questions may be regarded as the transition phase into intrusive questioning of the client.

1. How many times a day do you usually empty your bladder (urinate)?
2. Do you have any difficulty starting the stream?
3. Do you feel you empty the bladder completely every time?
4. Is there any dribbling? Burning?
5. Do you have to get up at night to empty your bladder? How often?
6. Has there been any change in the color or odor of the urine?
7. Do you have regular bowel movements? How often? What time of day?
8. Are the stools formed, brown, soft? Any change in color, consistency, frequency?
9. Do you take any medications for the bowels? What? Regularly? (Include hot water, prune juice, commercial laxatives, etc.)
10. Do you have hemorrhoids? Any medication? What? How often?

Sample History—Routine Yearly Physical

Following is an example of a client history demonstrating one method of recording the conversation. Only one part of the history is presented.

Name: Mr. A. B. Age: 34 Sex: Male
Height: 5′11″ (177 cm) Weight: 170# (77 kg) B.P. 130/76 Pulse: 72
Educational Accomplishments: College—M.A. Business Administration
Occupation: Vice-President City Bank

B. = Mr. A. B.   N. = Nurse who is interviewing

N. "Good morning Mr. B. How are you this morning?"
B. "Good morning. Fine, so far—if you don't find anything wrong with me."
N. (laughs) "Well, I hope everything's fine, too. My name is Mary Nelson. I work with Dr. C. I'm going to ask you some questions about your health history, and then Dr. C. will come in to examine you."
B. "O.K."
N. (Sits at desk—her chair is about three feet from where Mr. B. is seated.) "Are you comfortable?"
B. "Yes."

CARDIORESPIRATORY

N. "Do you ever have problems breathing?"
B. "No."
N. "Do you have any drainage from the nose or throat?"
B. "I have a little, first thing in the morning. But it clears up by breakfast."
N. "Do you have a chronic cough?"
B. "No. My wife says I have cigarette cough, but I don't agree."
N. "Do you smoke?"
B. "Yes."
N. "How many cigarettes?"
B. "About a pack a day—filters."
N. [Pick up on guilt feelings (filters) for use in planning teaching against smoking] "Pipe?"
B. "No."
N. "Marijuana?"
B. "No."

© 1977 Wiley

THE NURSING HISTORY

N. "Do you ever experience chest pain when breathing deeply?"
B. "No. Except when I've overdone on the jogging, I get short of breath for a few minutes. But then there's no pain after that."
N. "Is there a history of lung cancer, emphysema, T.B., COPD, or asthma in your family?"
B. "My father died of a heart attack when he was fifty-nine. And I had an uncle who had COPD. He died at about fifty. He never did take very good care of himself. I think he was an alcoholic, too."
N. "How many pillows do you use at night?" (Notice that the nurse avoided making any judgmental statement about the uncle with supposed alcohol abuse.)
B. "One."
N. "Do you get a cold more than once a year?"
B. "Not even that often."
N. "Do you have allergies that bring on skin rash, blotches?"
B. "I'm allergic to penicillin. I got some in the service, and I broke out in hives. I've never taken it since."
N. "When you had the allergic reaction, were there any other symptoms?"
B. "No."
N. "Do you have any birthmarks or scars?"
B. "Yes. An appendix scar from when I was nine years old. Oh, and a scar on my left upper arm, where I fell out of a tree and had to have stitches, when I was seven. That's all."
N. "Have you noticed any change in your hair?"
B. "No. I have some dandruff, but it's controlled with dandruff shampoo."
N. "Do you experience chest pain?"
B. "No."
N. "Have you ever had any problems with high blood pressure?" "No." "Circulation?" "No." "Blood clotting?" "No." "Palpitations?" "No."
N. "Is there a history of heart disease, stroke, clotting problems, or circulatory disease in your family?"
B. "Well, as I told you before, my dad died of a heart attack. My mother had varicose veins. But she never had to take any medicine or have them surgically repaired. I think my grandmother died of a stroke. She died when I was a kid, so I don't remember the details."

NUTRITION

N. "What are your special food likes?"
B. "Meat, any kind. And fish. And potatoes. Really, I like just about anything."
N. "Any dislikes, allergies?" (Note: There is a difference between the two.)
B. "I don't like liver or spinach. But I'm not allergic to them, or any food that I know of."
N. "Do you ever have any problems with chewing or swallowing?"
B. "No."
N. "Do you take any food supplements, such as vitamins?"
B. "No. My wife makes me take vitamin C when I get the cold or flu. But I don't take anything like that on a regular basis."
N. "How many glasses of water, juice, pop, coffee, and so forth, would you say you drink per day?"
B. "Oh, about five cups of coffee a day. And one glass of juice. And one or two bowls of soup, depending on what my wife makes for supper. And maybe three glasses of water, if I added up what I drink from the fountain."
N. "What about beer, wine or other liquor? (You need to ask people because they tend to forget that liquor is liquid intake.)
B. "Oh I forgot about that. I usually have one cocktail when I get home from work. And I drink socially."
N. "Socially?" (Try to pick up cues to possible alcohol abuse. Also note nonverbal behaviors when the client answers.)
B. "Two or three drinks at a party—maybe twice a month."

© 1977 Wiley

40 NURSING ASSESSMENT

PROGRESS CHECK

1. Relate Mr. B's smoking habits to his cough and nasal drainage. What questions could you ask to get more information in these areas?

2. Relate Mr. B's alcohol intake to definition of alcoholism. What further questions would you ask to get more information in this area? Does nutritional status indicate chronic alcoholism?

3. What would you do if Mr. B refused to answer any of your questions about alcohol intake?
   a. Classify him as an alcoholic.
   b. Stop questioning him on the subject.
   c. Apologize for embarrassing him.
   d. Relate back to alcoholic intake when asking questions on nutritional status, coping mechanisms, and achievement.

ANSWERS
1. Chronic cough and morning postnasal drip are often signs of excessive smoking, beginning lung-tissue damage. Ask about the amount, character, color, thickness of sputum to distinguish from sinus infection or pneumonia. Ask about the cough. Is it productive, painful, persistent? What helps (cough medicine)?
2. Questions: Do you feel you "need" the cocktail before dinner? Do you feel the need for drinking alcohol when you get up in the morning? Do you drink until you lose your memory? Do you drink to get over a hangover? Mr. B's nutritional status does not indicate chronic alcoholism.
3. b and d. Mr. B is not necessarily an alcoholic because he doesn't want to answer questions about alcohol intake. He may feel somewhat threatened by intrusive questioning. Avoid "labeling."

ACTIVITY 3

THE CLIENT HISTORY CONTENT: PSYCHO-SOCIOCULTURAL HUMAN NEEDS

SEXUALITY
This category of questions seeks to determine the client's feelings about himself as a person. Thus, the questions concern body image, feelings about sexual identity and self-concept, as well as physical genital status. This category is the transition from physical to psycho-sociocultural assessment, as it probes both areas. Some of the questions are quite sensitive and should be asked

© 1977 Wiley

with discretion. If your questioning is making the client uncomfortable, he may express it verbally, but more often you will see nonverbal cues. The client may avert his eyes, wring his hands, shift his position often, swing his leg, cross and uncross his arms and legs, or toy with an object, such as handkerchief, lighter, or pencil. If you observe these behaviors, you may do one of two things. First, you might ask the client if he is uncomfortable with the questions you are asking. Second, you might shift your inquiries to another subject, temporarily, and return to this questioning later. On the other hand, sometimes you may meet a client who has many queries and concerns in this area and is very glad that someone has finally given him the chance to get the desired information.

1. Male only: Are you experiencing any genital problems? Painful erection? Inability to culminate the sex act? Any unusual discharge from the penis? Any history of V.D.? Vasectomy? Any genital problems?

2. Female only: Gravida _____ Para _____ Abortions _____ Date of first menses _____ Regular _____ Pain with menses _____ Any vaginal discharge _____ Have your breasts changed in size or shape since your last physical exam? Do you do a self breast exam every month? Any history of V.D.? Birth control? Hysterectomy? Oopherectomy? Any genital problems?

3. Both male and female: Do you feel that your sexual life is adequate, fulfilling?

4. How do you feel about yourself as a man/woman? Pleased?

5. Parent: How do you feel about being a mother/father? Do you feel satisfied, adequate? Do you plan to have more children?

6. Do you think you get along well with other men/women?

Supplement
If there seem to be any abnormalities, either physical or psychological, further questioning is called for. Be sure to pick up any nonverbal cues that will help you assess the comfort or distress the client may be experiencing. Social taboos against discussing sexuality openly are not easily overcome, and cultural and religious overtones need to be considered. Culturally, most Americans are still secretive about sexuality because they believe it is a very private and personal subject. Also, some religions have very specific laws governing sexual practice (Catholic, Jewish, for example), and personal choices by persons of these faiths are nonexistent or minimized.

If the client appears very anxious, it may be necessary to postpone this section (or any section) or to restrict questions to physical assessment only. Hopefully, the client-nurse relationship could improve to the point where the subject can be continued. But don't be alarmed if this sometimes does not happen.

AFFILIATION
These questions should help you appraise the client's relationship to significant others, and to friends and associates.

1. Do you live alone? With others? How many people do you live with? (Nuclear or extended family)

2. Do you feel close ties with your family? Do you get along with the family members in your household?

3. Would you say you have a "happy" family? Tell me about it.

4. Who is the most important "other" in your life?

5. Does he/she live with you? Close to you?

6. Do you ever feel lonely? Tell me about it.

7. Do you constantly like or need people around you, or do you enjoy periods of aloneness?

8. Do you generally get along with the people with whom you work?

© 1977 Wiley

42 NURSING ASSESSMENT

9. Would you say that you are satisfied with most of your relationships with people? Are you generally well liked?
10. What is your religious affiliation?

ACHIEVEMENT
This set of questions attempts to ascertain the client's perception of his goals, immediate and long-range. Clues to self-motivation can be picked up here.

1. Can you describe your lifestyle for me? (Concept of work, success, motivators.)
2. If you had your choice, would you keep your present job, or change it? (If retired, talk about lifestyle.)
3. Do you like your job? Are you planning to continue, or move on to another? Do you fear losing your job?
4. Do you think you are making the kind of income you and your family can be happy with?
5. Do you feel you are important to your job? Family? Society?
6. Are you in a good mood most of the time? Have a good memory?

SAFETY
This section should help you assess both physical and psychological safety. Obtain a copy of a home-safety checklist. This can usually be obtained from a community health agency. Also, ascertain if the client has a safety program at work. This is the section in which you review any medications which the client takes.

1. Are you aware of keeping the home safe for yourself and your family? Keep appliances in good repair? Keep house and yard in good repair?
2. List all of the medications that are in your home. Do you know the actions, dosages, routes of administration, side-effects, antidotes?
3. Do you follow the prescription completely? Not administer the medication to any other family member without a doctor's order? Discard outdated medications? Store the medications out of reach of children? How do you store the medications? In the bottles with proper labels? Where are medicines kept for persons unable to open new types of bottles? (Elderly, arthritic.)
4. Do you feel secure in your family relationships? Do you feel able to protect your family?

Sample History, Continued: Mr. A.B.

The following example demonstrates part of the history of the client's needs of sexuality, achievement, affiliation, and safety.

SEXUALITY
    N. "Are you experiencing any genital problems?"
    B. "No."
    N. "Painful erection?" "No." "Inability to culminate the sexual act?" "No."
    N. "Any unusual discharge from the penis?"
    B. "No."
    N. "Any history of V.D.?"
    B. "I had gonorrhea in the army. That's when I got the penicillin and the reaction. But I haven't had any V.D. since."
    N. "Did you have a vasectomy?"
    B. "No."
    N. "Do you feel that your sexual life is adequate, fulfilling?"
    B. "Yes."

© 1977 Wiley

N. "How do you feel about yourself as a man?"
B. "O.K. I like myself the way I am." (Observe nonverbal behavior.)
N. "How do you feel about being a father?"
B. "Great! I have two kids, ages twelve and ten. They're the pride of my life. Oh sure, I have to discipline them once in a while, but on the whole, I think we're a pretty happy family."
N. "Do you plan to have more children?"
B. "No."
N. "Would you say that you get along well with other men?"
B. "Yes."
N. "Women?"
B. "Yes."
N. "How many people live in your house?"
B. "Just my wife, kids and me."
N. "From what you've already told me, you have pretty good relationships with your wife and children, right?"
B. "Oh yes. I think compared to a lot of families I know, we're very happy."

AFFILIATION
N. "Who is the most important "other" in your life?"
B. "My wife is my best friend. You know, they say the biggest reason for divorce that people give nowadays is that the partner has 'changed.' Well, my wife and I have both changed over the years, but we still like each other, and like doing things together."
N. "Do you ever feel lonely?"
B. "Not really. When I'm away from home on business, I call Sheila, my wife, and we have a nice visit. But it doesn't hurt to be alone once in a while. That's why I have my den at home."
N. "Do you generally get along with the people with whom you work?"
B. "Generally. I'm in charge of hiring and firing, though, and sometimes that gets a bit touchy. But on the whole, I'd say I get along with most of the people."
N. "Would you say that you get along with most people, aside from work?"
B. "Yes."
N. "What is your religious affiliation?"
B. "Protestant."

ACHIEVEMENT
N. "What is your concept of work related to success?"
B. "Hmmm. (pause) Well, I guess I'd say that success to me is being well enough to work and provide for my family, and have a few luxuries on the side."
N. "What motivates you to work?"
B. "Well, my family responsibilities. And I enjoy my work, too. I hope to be a bank president someday."
N. "Do you fear losing your job?"
B. "No."
N. "Do you think you're making the kind of income your family is happy with?"
B. "Yes. When I was in college, we had one kid, and it was pretty rough for a while. So now we appreciate what we have. Luckily, we're not caught in the 'keep up with the Joneses' game."
N. "Do you feel you are important to your job?"
B. "Yes."
N. "To your family?"
B. "Yes."
N. "To society?"
B. "Well, I hadn't thought of it that way, but I guess I am."
N. "Are you in a good mood most of the time?"
B. "Yeah. Except when the kids don't keep the house picked up, or they wake up their mother on Sunday morning." (Both laugh.)

© 1977 Wiley

44 NURSING ASSESSMENT

SAFETY

N. "Are you aware of keeping the home safe for yourself and your family?"
B. "Yes. I'm somewhat of a handyman, and I fix frayed cords and small appliances. And my wife calls the repairman if any big thing happens. My neighbor got into a big lawsuit because he had a hole in his sidewalk, and some lady tripped in it and broke her hip. So, I'm pretty conscious of keeping things in good repair."
N. "Tell me all the medications that are in your home right now."
B. "Well, let's see. There's aspirin, and Alka-Seltzer, oh, and my wife's birth-control pills, and vitamin C."
N. "Do you know the actions and dosages of all these medications?"
B. "Yes. My wife told me about the BC pills. And I know about the others."
N. "Do you know the side-effects and antidotes for these medicines?"
B. "Yes. Besides, we have the number for the poison-control center right beside the telephone."
N. "Do you feel able to protect your family from external dangers?"
B. "Reasonably. They know what to do in case of fire. And we have our house and possessions insured."

PROGRESS CHECK

1. List the eight basic needs of man. Classify them as four predominantly physical-cultural and four predominantly psycho-sociocultural.

2. Write an outline of important questions (three in each category) to ask when taking a client history.

3. Write down the responses *you* would give in Activity 3. Note your feelings about writing them down. Relate your feelings to those the clients may have about giving such information to you.

© 1977 Wiley

4. Take a nursing history from three classmates and two friends or relatives.

ANSWERS

1. *Physical-cultural*   *Psycho-sociocultural*

   Activity—Rest   Sexuality
   Nutrition   Affiliation
   Elimination   Achievement
   Cardiorespiration   Safety

2. Activity—Rest (sleep pattern, ADL, recreational patterns)
   Nutrition (diet history, cultural implications, allergies)
   Elimination (pattern of stool elim., pattern of urine elim., what causes change in pattern)
   Cardiorespiration (any cardiac problems, any respiratory problems, smoking habits)
   Sexuality (normal anatomy, physiology of sex organs, self-image)
   Achievement (job satisfaction, goals—immediate, long-range)
   Affiliation (family relationships, friends, associates)
   Safety (physical, home, recreation, job, psychological)

ACTIVITY 4
THE CLIENT HISTORY CONTENT: COPING MECHANISMS

Whenever a person experiences an alteration in input, he or she needs to make an adjustment. The adjustment may be physical or psychological, or both. The method of coping may vary, depending on the nature and severity of the alteration. The purpose of this series of questions is to assess the usual mechanisms by which clients are able to adjust themselves, and to ascertain the effectiveness of the mechanism.

1. When you are confronted with a problem, how do you usually handle it? Do you make an assessment of the problem?
2. Do you explore alternatives for solving the problem?
3. Do you:
   a. Share the problem with anyone?
   b. Become very anxious? What happens when you are anxious?
   c. Become angry? Take it out on someone, something?
   d. Get depressed?
   e. Try to blame someone? Yourself? Others?
   f. Drink? Get drunk?
   g. Try to forget that there is a problem?
   h. Get a headache? Stomach ache? Diarrhea?
   i. Pray for guidance to solve the problem?
4. Are you able to make a decision, and once you've made it, stick to it?
5. Are you able to accept the decision, once you've made it, and stick to it?
6. Do you feel that most of the time you've made correct decisions?

Supplement

What you are really doing here is assessing the client's ability to solve problems. If the client needs something concrete to discuss, you may pose such changes as financial crisis, birth, death, or injury. The problem may be hypothetical or real.

© 1977 Wiley

Sample History, Continued: Mr. A.B.

The following example demonstrates part of the history of the client's coping mechanisms.

N. "When you are faced with a problem, do you try to define the problem?"
B. "Yes. We learned how important this is in graduate school."
N. "Do you usually explore alternatives to solving the problem, or jump to a solution right away?"
B. "Usually, if I'm angry, I try to get myself calmed down first. Then I attack the problem. A couple of weeks ago, my ten-year-old son came home with news that some older kid was selling pep-pills near the playground. I was furious, and my first instinct was to go right over there and kill him. But then I went into my study and sat and thought for a while. Then, I came up with some alternative plans of action."
N. "Go on."
B. "I called the principal of the school, and a couple of other parents whom I knew would want to be in on the meeting, and arranged to get together and talk out the whole problem. I knew it was something I couldn't solve myself."
N. "And this is how you usually tackle a problem?"
B. "Yes. Of course, if it's a family problem, we keep it in the family. My wife and I are pretty together on our thinking, and we solve problems pretty much to both our satisfaction."
N. "It sounds like you share your problems. Do you ever take out your anger on something or someone?"
B. "No. I usually retreat to reconnoiter."
N. "Do you get easily depressed over a problem?"
B. "No."
N. "Do you find yourself blaming?"
B. "It depends. Sometimes."
N. "Do you get drunk?"
B. "No."
N. "Do you try to forget there is a problem?"
B. "No."
N. "Get a headache, or other symptoms?"
B. "No."
N. "Pray?"
B. "Sometimes."
N. "Are you able to make a decision on how to handle or solve a problem?"
B. "Most of the time. For instance, when our concerned group met about the drug problem, we came up with a couple of solutions, and I was able to accept the final decision."
N. "Do you follow through on most of your decisions?"
B. "Yes. A good example of this is when one of the kids needs to be punished for doing something wrong. My wife and I come to a decision, and we both stick to it."
N. "Do you feel that most of the time you make the right decisions?"
B. "Yes."

PROGRESS CHECK

1. Of the alternative behaviors listed under *Coping Mechanisms,* which are functional and which are nonfunctional?

© 1977 Wiley

2. List the coping behaviors you use. Relate these behaviors to functional, nonfunctional behavior.

3. Identify the coping behaviors of five persons by means of history-taking.
4. Ask two people: "If you broke a leg this afternoon, and were hospitalized for five days, how would you deal with the problem?" Record the responses and compare the coping mechanisms used.

ACTIVITY 5
THE CLIENT HISTORY CONTENT: ALTERATIONS IN INPUT

The first part of the history of a person with an alteration in input is essentially the same as in Activities 2 and 3. However, when interviewing this type of client, you will want to begin the questioning with the immediate problem for which the client has sought help. This problem is his chief concern, and your interest in it will probably elicit his cooperation in seeking the rest of the history. If the problem is directly related to any of the sections already recorded above, then utilize that section out of order to help you assess the immediate problem.

Following are some categories of alterations of input. Death and dying are extremely important to learn how to deal with, and an excellent book has been written on the subject by Elisabeth Kubler-Ross. Please refer to her writings (especially Chapters 3–8) for assessment techniques.

ILLNESS AND PAIN
Illness and pain are dealt with together, because the purpose is to assess pain and illness that is not readily and easily dealt with by the client, and for which he is seeking medical attention.

1. Describe the pain for me.
2. Where is the pain? (Local, radiating, diffuse?).
3. Is the pain dull, sharp, heavy, throbbing, stabbing, burning, deep, peripheral, continuous, or intermittent?
4. What makes the pain worse?
5. Does anything help ease the pain?
6. How long does the pain last?
7. How long have you had this problem? Have you ever been hospitalized for it?
8. Have you had any previous hospitalizations for any other problem? Any surgeries?

© 1977 Wiley

48 NURSING ASSESSMENT

ANXIETY, DEPRESSION
1. You seem worried (depressed). Can you tell me about it?
2. Do you feel unable to cope with this problem?

Supplement
You need to decide quickly if this client is in need of psychological intervention. If you pick up any clues that he is not in full touch with reality, or that anxiety seems to be prohibiting his carrying out activities of daily living, then a more comprehensive psychiatric examination is in order.

LOSS, GRIEVING
The purpose of questioning in this area is to ascertain the level of grief at which the client seems to be functioning. Loss in this section does not refer to death and dying, but to illness, hospitalization, and surgery.

1. How do you feel about being in the hospital? Confined to bed?
2. Do you understand your treatments? Operation?
3. How do you feel about it? Frightened? Worried? Angry? Sad? Hopeful?
4. Do you feel you can adjust to the results of the operation? (Refers to anatomical change, sensory loss.)
5. Do you have trust in your doctors? Nurses? Technicians?

POVERTY
Questions in this area may refer to an existing economic situation that has been long-lasting, or to a situation caused by temporary or permanent loss of wages because of illness and/or hospitalization. Again, much sensitivity is needed here, because this is a very delicate subject to most people.

1. Are you usually able to pay your bills?
2. Do you usually have enough food at home? Heat? Electricity? Water?
3. Do you have a job? Are you able to return to your previous employment after this hospitalization?
4. Do you have medical insurance? Do you need help to pay this (clinic, hospital) bill? Would you like to talk to a social worker?

TERMINATING THE INTERVIEW
Always remember that client comfort is more important than your information-gathering task. If the client is in physical or emotional stress, limit the questions and resume inquiries at a later time. Many times, stress is expressed nonverbally by unfriendly facial expression, increased hand movements, and even body positioning (turning away from the interviewer).

At the conclusion of the interview, tell the client that you have finished the questioning. Ask if he wishes to add anything. Thank the client for the time and cooperation. Assure the client that the information will be used to help plan for good care. Leave with a reminder that if any information is remembered that might be important, to contact you, and you will be glad to supplement your data.

Sample History: An Ill Woman Who Has Been Hospitalized Today

This history is written out, for the most part, in a narrative report style. The interviewer collected the data and then wrote the narrative. Note that the most apparent problems are dealt with at the beginning of the interview.

© 1977 Wiley

BASIC INFORMATION

Name: Mrs. C. R. Age: 69 Sex: Female
Height: 150 cm (approx.) Weight: 90# (40.9 kg) B.P.: 190/110
Pulse: 96 Educational Accomplishments: Eighth grade
Occupation: Homemaker

CARDIORESPIRATORY

Usually, Mrs. R. has no trouble breathing. But four nights ago she noticed that she had to use three pillows (as opposed to the usual two—due to kyphosis) in order to get her breath. Breathing became more shallow and labored and this was the reason her daughter-in-law brought her to the doctor. She usually has no drainage from nose or throat. But now she has developed a productive cough. She also has a great deal of chest pain.

Mrs. R. does not smoke and never has. Her sister died of pneumonia when she was a baby. There are no other familial respiratory problems. Mrs. R. has had pneumonia three times in the last four years. She has been hospitalized twice. She has no known allergies that present respiratory symptoms. She has no scars or birthmarks. Her hair is very thin. There is no sign of dermatological problems.

Mrs. R. has been a known hypertensive for fifteen years and has been fairly under control. She is somewhat forgetful about taking the medications regularly. This has been remedied for five years since moving in with her family. She is presently on Aldomet, hydrochlorthiazide, and potassium chloride. Apparently she has no overt cardiac problems. She says her ECG's have always been normal for a woman her age. She denies clotting problems, palpitations, or a racing heart. Her mother and father both died of strokes in old age. Her brother died of a heart attack, and she has a sister who has hypertension.

ELIMINATION

Mrs. R. usually has a bowel movement every other morning. She is very prone to constipation and sometimes takes milk-of-magnesia (about three times a week). She never has problems with diarrhea. She has hemorrhoids but they don't bother her too much. She doesn't take medication for them.

Mrs. R. urinates three or four times a day and usually two or three times at night. She has a little difficulty starting the stream but feels she empties the bladder completely, if she "gives herself enough time." There was no dribbling or burning up until about four days ago, when she began to have burning and some frequency and dribbling. The urine has become darker yellow and more odorous.

ACTIVITY

Mrs. R. is a chronically ill woman, who has just been readmitted for hypertension, pneumonia, and urinary tract infection. She lives with her son and daughter-in-law and four grandchildren. She spends most of the day in a large overstuffed chair in the family room. Because of arthritis, her activities are greatly curtailed. She feels frustrated that she cannot be of more help around the house. Her day usually begins at about 7:00 when she arises. She feels the most energy early in the morning, so she gets dressed and eats breakfast. Then she putters around the kitchen doing dishes, and in the flower room taking care of a large collection of potted plants. After lunch she naps for an hour or two, then retires to the family room. When the children come home from school, they join her in the family room and fill her in on the day's activities. She eats supper with the family, then retires for the night. She usually gets up to the bathroom two or three times a night. During the last three nights she has been up almost every hour and now feels exhausted. She usually gets about ten to twelve hours of sleep per twenty-four, except the last few days when she had to get up so often at night. Up until a few days ago she has felt rested when arising in the morning.

Mrs. R. wears glasses for reading, but has very poor eyesight. She has full dentures, which fit well. She has impaired movement: she walks very slowly with the help of a cane. She is stooped and she winces when sitting down or arising. She does not have uncoordinated movements.

© 1977 Wiley

COPING MECHANISMS

Mrs. R. says that when she is faced with a problem she usually confides in her daughter-in-law. She also believes strongly in the power of prayer and resorts to prayer very soon after the problem appears. She says that when she was younger she would develop nausea whenever there was a serious problem, but that doesn't happen any more. She tends to blame the devil for the evil that exists and also for problems that arise within the family. She believes that illness is a test from God to see if a person has enough faith. She says that her daughter-in-law usually lets her try to solve the problem, but does offer advice. An example of this is when Timmy, the oldest grandchild, would come home late at night and park underneath her window. This always awakened her and she had a hard time getting back to sleep. She talked it over with her daughter-in-law, and then with Timmy. Timmy agreed to park on the other side of the house and the problem was resolved.

ILLNESS AND PAIN

Mrs. R. says she is having a great deal of chest pain. She describes it as constant, dull, aching, deep pain. Taking a deep breath and talking and moving around makes the pain worse. Lying very still makes it feel better. The pain began about four days ago and has gotten worse. She had the same problem three times before and was hospitalized twice.

Mrs. R. also has dysuria. She says she has trouble starting the stream and then experiences sharp, burning pain. It stops when she stops the stream. The dysuria began a few days ago. She's never had this problem before.

LOSS, HOSPITALIZATION

Mrs. R. does not mind being in the hospital, because "I know the doctors and nurses will help me and I'm too sick to stay at home." She hates the thought of IPPB and percussion and postural drainage, but she is resigned because she knows they will help her. She knows they are going to take a lot of blood samples and urine tests and she perceives them as necessary, so she doesn't resist. She is a little sad that she has to be away from her family, but she knows they will come to visit often. She says she trusts and respects the doctors and nurses. She would like two things: a third pillow and a warm glass of milk at bedtime. She does not think that she is going to die but says she has no fear of death—she can join her husband.

This interview was done in three segments in order to give Mrs. R. the chance to rest from the exertion of talking. There are many clues for planning the care of Mrs. R. in this history; thus, it fulfills the requirements for a comprehensive tool.

PROGRESS CHECK

1. Take a client history from five persons who are experiencing one or more alterations in input. Try to include one person who is dying, and one baby.
2. Record two client histories, using the two methods demonstrated in Activities 2, 3, 4, and 5.
3. Write out a list of questions you would include in the history of a 12-month-old baby, taken from the mother.

ANSWERS

In order to take a client history on an infant or child, refer to a pediatrics textbook for variations in needs and problems at the differing age levels. Find a reliable history-giver, such as parent or guardian, babysitter, or friend of the family.

a. Activity—nap times, toys related to age, indoor/outdoor activities, crawling, walking.
b. Cardiorespiratory—prone to "colds," "flu," allergies, anomalies (congenital heart, etc.), tonsillitis, bruising or bleeding.

© 1977 Wiley

c. Nutrition—formula (include amount), foods related to age, eating habits, digestive problems, allergies, regurgitation, weight-for-age.
d. Elimination—how many diapers/day, consistency, color amount, number/day of stool.
e. Sexuality—dress in male/female clothes, call by name.
f. Affiliation—cuddling, holding, words or expressions used to convey meaning, acceptance by other family members, sibling rivalry.
g. Safety—crib, surroundings (cupboards, medicine chests, cleaning agents, wall plugs, cords, paint and plaster, garbage disposal), reliable babysitter, clothing.
h. Coping mechanisms—anxiety, anger, unusual crying behavior, withdrawal, unusual fear, vomiting that is persistent or associated with other psychological manifestations.

SUMMARY

The areas of inquiry for a client interview have been presented systematically. It cannot be emphasized enough that you must internalize and tailor the material to make it your own. The client interview should be relaxed and informal. Practice interviewing your friends until you come up with questions in the phrases with which you are most comfortable. In other words, use your own language. You should try to memorize as much of the interview content as possible in order to focus your undivided attention on the client and what he is saying, verbally and nonverbally.

POSTTEST

1. A client history:
   a. may be taken by any nursing personnel
   b. is the same as a nursing history
   c. need not be taken on well persons
   d. should be taken by an R.N. or nursing student
      1. a and b
      2. a and c
      3. b and d
      4. c and d

2. The client history is *not* a:
   a. medical history
   b. process of gathering facts about a client's coping behavior
   c. nursing data base
   d. a tool for determining interventions for nursing care
      1. a and b
      2. a and d
      3. b and c
      4. c and d

Mrs. Diaz is an 81-year-old Mexican-American woman admitted one hour ago with a diagnosis of fractured hip. She speaks Spanish only. She appears frightened and in a great deal of pain. The following five questions refer to Mrs. Diaz.

3. Elements of the internal environment of Mrs. Diaz are:
   a. pain
   b. fear
   c. nationality

© 1977 Wiley

52 NURSING ASSESSMENT

    d. fracture
       1. a and b
       2. a and d
       3. b and c
       4. c and d

4. Before beginning the history you can establish a climate of trust with Mrs. Diaz by:
   a. assuring her that everything will be all right
   b. getting an order for relief of pain
   c. speaking Spanish or getting an interpreter
   d. giving her your undivided attention
   1. a and b
   2. b, c, and d
   3. none of the above
   4. all of the above

5. Which are Mrs. Diaz' basic needs?
   a. sexuality, achievement
   b. affiliation
   c. safety
   d. cardiorespiratory, nutrition, elimination
   1. d only
   2. b and c
   3. all except a
   4. all of the above

6. Because Mrs. Diaz is anxious and in pain, which of the following can be delayed until a later time?
   a. history of how the fracture was sustained
   b. name of her closest living relative
   c. vital signs
   d. assessment of dietary habits
   1. b only
   2. d only
   3. a and d
   4. none of the above

Peter Jones is a five-year-old boy who has come to the clinic for a preschool checkup, accompanied by his mother. The following five questions pertain to Peter.

7. The nursing history should be taken:
   a. by the doctor
   b. by the nurse
   c. from Peter's mother only
   d. from Peter and his mother together
   1. a and c
   2. a and d
   3. b and c
   4. b and d

8. A client history from Peter will:
   a. determine his eating habits
   b. rule out diabetes and heart disease
   c. identify any medications he takes
   1. b only
   2. a and c
   3. all of the above

© 1977 Wiley

9. Appropriate questions to ask of Peter are:
   a. What kinds of games do you like to play?
   b. If someone at school offers you a pill, will you take it?
   c. Who is your best friend?
   d. How many hours of sleep do you get?
      1. a and c
      2. a and d
      3. b and c
      4. b and d

10. Of the following, which are Peter's basic needs:
    a. nurturance
    b. fairly regular elimination pattern
    c. male and female identity figures
    d. achievement, motivation
       1. a and b
       2. b, c, and d
       3. none of the above
       4. all of the above

11. The following coping mechanisms have been identified. Which are abnormal for Peter's age and require further assessment?
    a. aggression
    b. fantasy friends
    c. enuresis
    d. thumb sucking
       1. a and b
       2. a and d
       3. b and c
       4. c and d

Mr. Sanders is a 50-year-old married man admitted with the history of gastric distress. He is going to have tests to determine the presence of an ulcer. The following questions pertain to Mr. Sanders.

12. You are about to begin the client history when Mr. Sanders says, "I'm really worried about the tests I'm going to have." What would be your best action?
    a. Begin the history with the section on anxiety.
    b. Say, "There's nothing to worry about, the tests are not painful."
    c. Ask, "Worried? Would you like to tell me about it?"
    d. Remind him that you have a time limit to get the history done.
       1. a and b
       2. a and c
       3. b and d
       4. c and d

13. During the interview you learn that Mr. Sanders is worried about his job. What would your next action be?
    a. Change the subject.
    b. Relate his guilt feelings to the gastric pain.
    c. Obtain the information matter-of-factly.
    d. Say, "They can't fire you after all the years you've put in."
       1. a only
       2. c only
       3. b and d
       4. b, c, and d

© 1977 Wiley

14. Of the following nonverbal behavior, which would give you clues that Mr. Sanders may be apprehensive about your questions?
    a. averting his eyes
    b. wincing with pain
    c. crossing and uncrossing his legs every two to three minutes
    d. twisting a rubber band until it breaks
       1. a and b
       2. all except b
       3. all except c
       4. none of the above

15. Of the following history areas, which ones should be covered more carefully with Mr. Sanders?
    a. cardiorespiratory
    b. nutrition, elimination
    c. safety
    d. activity, rest
       1. a and b
       2. a and d
       3. b and c
       4. b and d

16. When you question Mr. Sanders about the pain, which of the following are appropriate?
    a. When did you first notice the particular pain?
    b. Is the pain intermittent or continuous?
    c. Describe the pain.
    d. What do you do to relieve the pain?
       1. c only
       2. a, b, and c
       3. b, c, and d
       4. all of the above

17. Mrs. Sanders enters the room during your history gathering. What action should you take?
    a. Include her in your questioning.
    b. Introduce yourself to her.
    c. Ask her to wait in the lounge for a few minutes.
    d. Go on with your questions, ignoring her.
       1. d only
       2. a and b
       3. b anc c
       4. none of the above

18. Listed below are six categories that are used when taking a client history. For each category, state one question that would be specific for obtaining information from a 10-year-old healthy girl:
    a. activity—rest

    b. nutrition

    c. safety

© 1977 Wiley

d. affiliation

e. achievement

f. sexuality

Answers

1. 3	6. 2	11. 1	16. 4
2. 2	7. 4	12. 2	17. 3
3. 1	8. 3	13. 2	
4. 2	9. 1	14. 2	
5. 4	10. 4	15. 1	

18. a. activity—rest (pattern sometimes altered during growth spurts, games, and sports)
    b. nutrition (fad foods, school lunches and snacks)
    c. safety (bicycles, skates, other toys, safety while playing games, where games are played, feelings of safety with family, peers, and drugs at school)
    d. affiliation (relationship with parents, siblings, peers, teachers, clubs like Girl Scouts, Campfire Girls, and so forth, and school environment)
    e. achievement (school work-attitude, attention, memory, and competitiveness)
    f. sexuality (self-concept, sex role identification)

References

Roe, Anne K.; Sherwood, Mary C.; and Dunham, Frances, Nursing Communication Skills. New York: John Wiley & Sons, 1975.

© 1977 Wiley

GLORIA C. SCHMIDT R.N., M.N.

WILEY NURSING CONCEPT MODULE

PHYSICAL HEALTH ASSESSMENT

CONTENTS

    PRETEST 59   Answers 62

    INTRODUCTION 65

    TERMINAL OBJECTIVES 65

        ACTIVITY 1. Health History 67
        ACTIVITY 2. Physical Examination 67
        ACTIVITY 3. Inspection 71
        ACTIVITY 4. Palpation 72
        ACTIVITY 5. Percussion 74
        ACTIVITY 6. Auscultation 76
        ACTIVITY 7. Developing a Statement of Physical Health Assessment 77

    POSTTEST 81   Answers 84

    REFERENCES AND SUGGESTED READINGS 86

© 1977 Wiley

PRETEST

The Pretest is divided into two parts. Part A is a mixture of objective and discussion questions. The student can evaluate and score these questions using the Pretest answers. Part B has demonstration questions that must be performed for and evaluated by an instructor or perceptor using the guidelines stated in the answers.

Part A   Circle the *letter* indicating the correct answer on all multiple-choice questions. Answer all other questions as directed. Each question is worth one point unless otherwise indicated.

1. Some of the following are the steps in a logical sequential format for a physical examination. Place the numbers 1, 2, 3, etc. in the blanks to put the steps in sequence. Not all blanks need to be used. (4 points)
   ____temperature, pulse, respiration, blood pressure
   ____blood pressure, heart, lungs, breasts, axillae, abdomen, genitalia, extremities
   ____head, neck, back, posterior chest
   ____head, neck, heart, lungs, breast, axillae
   ____abdomen, back, posterior chest, genitalia, rectum/pelvic
   ____rectal or pelvic and rectal examination

2. Choose one of the above steps and state a rationale for its order. (2 points)

3. Describe three types of data that should be obtained from auscultation of the thorax and lungs. (6 points)

4. Match the following descriptions of observations with the area of general inspection. Letters may be used more than once. (6 points)

   Observation   *Area of Inspection*

   ____lying on side, splinting chest   a. body features
   ____paralysis of left side   b. state of consciousness
   ____alert, responsive   c. speech
   ____cyanosis of fingers and nails   d. body movement
   ____incoherent   e. outstanding signs
   ____rapid tremor of left hand

5. What depth is meant by the term "deep palpation"?
   a. 4 millimeters
   b. 1 inch
   c. 4 centimeters
   d. until resistance is met

6. List three observations that would be made by palpation of the anterior chest. (3 points)

© 1977 Wiley

60 NURSING ASSESSMENT

7. List five characteristics of a palpable mass that should be described. (5 points)

8. Match the body area with the sound elicited on percussion. The letters may be used more than once. (6 points)
   ____ normal lung
   ____ liver
   ____ gas-filled stomach
   ____ thigh
   ____ lung on deep inspiration
   ____ heart

   a. tympany
   b. hyperresonance
   c. resonance
   d. dullness
   e. flatness

9. What is the significance of dullness heard when percussing the flank area?

10. The stethoscope with the diaphragm headpiece allows which type sounds to be transmitted?
    a. all sounds
    b. low-pitched sounds
    c. medium-pitched sounds
    d. high-pitched sounds

11. In what areas of the neck should auscultation be used? Indicate the *letter* that gives the correct combination of responses.
    1. over the parotid glands
    2. over the carotid arteries
    3. over the thyroid gland
    4. over the muscles

    a. 1 and 4
    b. 2 and 3
    c. 3 and 4
    d. 1, 2, 3

12. Match the following descriptions with the correct type of breath sound. (3 points)
    ____ normally heard over the trachea; expiratory note is longer than inspiratory and there is a separation between the phases
    ____ normal breath sound heard when lung tissue overlies the large bronchi
    ____ breath sounds in which the inspiratory phase is longer and stronger than expiratory phase

    a. asthmatic
    b. vesicular
    c. bronchial
    d. bronchovesicular

13. Match the descriptions in the left list with the auscultatory valve areas in the right list. (4 points)
    ____ 5th left interspace, mid-clavicular line
    ____ 2nd right interspace at the sternal border
    ____ 2nd left interspace just lateral to sternum
    ____ 4th or 5th interspace, just left of sternum or at junction of sternum and xiphoid process

    a. aortic area
    b. pulmonic area
    c. mitral area
    d. tricuspid area

14. When examining the abdomen, which of the following should be done after inspection?
    a. review laboratory findings
    b. palpation
    c. percussion
    d. auscultation

© 1977 Wiley

PHYSICAL HEALTH ASSESSMENT **61**

15. Mr. King comes to you with the complaint of a harsh cough of one week's duration. Describe how you would assess this respiratory complaint, including the following in your description:
    a. initial observations to be made by a general inspection while listening to the client's description of the complaint

    b. information to be obtained about the present illness for the history

    c. data related to examination of the thorax and lungs to be gathered when using each of the following four techniques: inspection, palpation, percussion, auscultation

    d. how to use the data to formulate an assessment statement (12 points—3 for each part)

Part B The following must be performed for and evaluated by an instructor or preceptor using the guidelines for evaluation in the pretest answers. The student will demonstrate the skills called for in the objectives on palpation, percussion, and auscultation.

© 1977 Wiley

62 NURSING ASSESSMENT

16. You are given a sponge block model containing a mass. Palpate the mass and write a description of it, as you would if you were describing an anatomical mass. (5 points)

17. Using a manikin or classmate, demonstrate for your instructor or preceptor the proper techniques for palpation and bimanual percussion of the posterior chest. Include the following in your demonstration:
    a. systematic method of palpation, including:
        1. respiratory expansion (4 points)
        2. vocal fremitus (4 points)
    b. systematic method of bimanual or indirect percussion of the lungs (4 points)
18. Using a manikin or classmate, demonstrate for your instructor or preceptor correct auscultation of any *two* of the following:
    a. the anterior chest for heart sounds
    b. the anterior and posterior chest for breath sounds
    c. the abdomen (6 points–3 for each part demonstrated)

Answers

Part A

1. <u>1</u> temperature, pulse, respiration, BP
   <u>3</u> BP, heart, lungs, breasts, axillae, abdomen, genitalia, extremities
   <u>2</u> head, neck, back, posterior chest
   __ head, neck, heart, lungs, breasts, axillae
   __ abdomen, back, posterior chest, genitalia, rectum/pelvic
   <u>4</u> rectal or pelvic and rectal examination

2. Rationale for order of steps:
   Steps 1 and 2—Client is sitting upright, facilitating eye contact with examiner, ease of access to these parts, and comparison of physiological function when position is changed.
   Step 3—Examination and evaluation of all the body parts in this step is facilitated by the client's recumbent position.
   Step 4—Sufficient time has been allowed for rapport to be established and client cooperation gained.

3. a. character of breath sounds
   b. character of voice sounds
   c. presence or absence of any of the following: rales, wheezes, rhonchi, friction rub

4. a, a, b, e, c, d

5. c

6. Any three of the following: skin turgor, areas of tenderness, crepitation, thrills, pulsations, fremitus, friction rub, apical impulse, heaves, masses

7. Any five of the following: Location, shape, size, consistency, regularity of borders, mobility, tenderness

© 1977 Wiley

8. c, d, a, e, b, d
9. Dullness in the flank area could be an indication of fluid in the abdominal cavity.
10. d
11. b
12. c, d, b
13. c, a, b, d
14. d
15. Answer Guidelines: The student may use the symptom from the chief complaint to illustrate and describe the process or may simply describe the process and information to be gathered, as is done here.

    The process of assessment of a complaint is as follows:
    a. As the client describes the complaint initially, observe carefully the data described as the General Inspection—body features, state of consciousness, speech, body movement and outstanding signs, especially those which are associated with and verify the complaint. (any three of these must be stated or illustrated in the answer.)
    b. Interview the client to gather specific data about the complaint, including the kinds of information that would be gathered for the "Present Illness" part of a health history (any three of these four points must be stated or illustrated in the answer):
        1. an elaboration of the chief complaint with symptom characteristics—character, location, intensity or severity, timing, aggravating and relieving factors, associated symptoms
        2. history of the present problem—date and manner of onset, precipitating and predisposing factors related to onset
        3. description of the present status of the problem—course since onset; incidence or occurrences of symptom; progress—better, worse, unchanged; effect of any therapy
        4. summary of all significant positives and negatives related to the symptom
    c. Examine the client to gather physical signs, especially related to the thorax and lungs (at least three observations must be stated for each technique):
        1. inspection—configuration, symmetry, skin color, scars, pigmentation, lesions, character of respiratory movements
        2. palpation—temperature, texture, moisture of skin; fremitus, extent and symmetry of respiratory expansion, masses, tenderness
        3. percussion—symmetry of sound, abnormal sounds, boundaries of thoracic cavity, diaphragmatic excursion
        4. auscultation—character of breath and voice sounds, presence of rales, wheezes, rhonchi, friction rub
    d. To formulate an assessment statement (all three steps must be stated or illustrated):
        1. Tabulate all data and construct a logical report or record, eliminating irrelevant material and condensing relevant findings.
        2. Compare the summarized tabulated data with a known body of knowledge, such as obtained from textbooks, experts, and experience.
        3. Write a statement or statements that reflect the degree of correspondence between the client's findings and the known patterns of health and disease. This is the assessment statement.

Part B

16. Answer Guidelines: The description of the "mass" must include at least five of the following types of data: location (may use points of reference such as the part of a quadrant, clockface, or distance from the borders of the model), size (in centimeters), shape, consistency, regularity of borders, mobility, and tenderness.

© 1977 Wiley

64 NURSING ASSESSMENT

17. a. systematic method of palpation:
   1. Palpating respiratory expansion (must demonstrate at least four of the following):
      a. Warm hands.
      b. Use both hands simultaneously and palpate symmetrical areas of thorax.
      c. May use fingertips, palm, or ulnar edge of hand, but touch is applied lightly.
      d. Palpate from above down during normal and deep respiration.
      e. Should evaluate the degree and symmetry of expansion with respiration.
   2. Vocal fremitus (4 points as indicated):
      a–c. Steps a, b, and c are same as above (1 point).
      d. Ask client to repeat a resonant phrase—"1, 2, 3" or "99," etc. (1 point).
      e. Evaluates all lung segments from above down (1 point).
      f. Should evaluate comparative increase, decrease or absence (1 point).
   b. systematic method of percussion of the lungs:
   1. indirect percussion (must demonstrate at least four of the following):
      a. Press middle finger of left hand firmly against chest wall in intercostal spaces parallel to ribs. Other fingers on hand should not touch chest wall.
      b. Use middle finger of right hand to strike the base of the distal phalanx of finger on chest.
      c. Striking motion must be wrist action; forearm should be stationary. The blow should be quick and sharp.
      d. Chest should be percussed from side to side sequentially from the suprascapular area downward to lung base.
      e. Should identify the tone quality and describe density of underlying thoracic structures.

18. Evaluation guideline for heart sounds, breath sounds, and abdomen—auscultation demonstrations:
   1. Heart sounds (must include b, c, and d in demonstration):
      a. Ask client to hold breath while listening.
      b. Start with bell.
      c. Leave chestpiece at each auscultatory valve site for 3–4 seconds, listening in this order: (1) aortic area, (2) pulmonic area, (3) apex or mitral area, (4) tricuspid area.
      d. Repeat pattern using the diaphragm.
   2. Breath sounds on posterior and anterior chest (must include c, d, e):
      a. Have client seated.
      b. Tell client to breathe deeply through mouth; demonstrate this.
      c. Use diaphragm headpiece on stethoscope.
      d. Begin on posterior chest at *base* of lungs and work across upward, comparing symmetrical areas on both sides until reaching apex of lungs. Use this pattern:

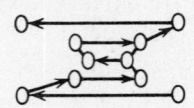

      e. Repeat same on anterior chest using similar pattern.
   3. The abdomen (must include all three):
      a. Know to auscultate before palpation or percussion.
      b. Use diaphragm.
      c. Listen in all four quadrants and is consistent in using a systematic pattern.

EVALUATION OF ANSWERS FOR SCORING

Part A: Total of 56 points is possible on Part A of the Pretest. A total of *44* points must be correct; in addition, answers to questions 10–14 must be correct to meet criteria stated in objectives.

Part B: Total of *15* points is possible for the demonstrations; *all* of these points must be earned.

© 1977 Wiley

INTRODUCTION

Assessment of a client's physical health involves gathering information in a variety of ways, such as (1) observing the client for strengths and weaknesses, (2) interviewing the client to obtain further information about strengths and weaknesses, (3) using a tactile approach, such as palpation during a physical examination, and (4) employing mechanical or technical assistance, such as an ECG and laboratory tests. In order to attach significance to the information gathered in these various ways, we must compare it to established standards of health. Conclusions drawn from these comparisons comprise the health assessment. From the health assessment, health problems can be identified and a plan of action formulated by the health professionals most capable of helping the client with each problem.

Sometimes nurses and paramedical personnel find that the data they gather through interacting with the client are not used by other health professionals. Clients also complain that several professionals may obtain the same data over and over and just put them in on a different form. It is this author's opinion that if nurses, doctors, and other health professionals use the same data base from which to formulate assessments, all could contribute to this base with data gathered at each client interaction, eliminating both of the above problems.

The medical history and physical examination formats are somewhat standardized and, in their unabbreviated state, cover a person's physical and psychosocial aspects, including the events of a typical day. Since the history and physical formats are accepted by the medical profession as a data base, and since they are certainly familiar to the nurse and others on the health team, it seems logical and expedient for nurses and paramedical personnel to contribute to and utilize these as the data base for a client's health assessment. Therefore, in this module on physical health assessment, the student will learn what data are needed for a physical examination as part of a physical health assessment, a systematic approach to gathering the data, some of the skills related to physical examination, such as inspection, palpation, percussion, and auscultation; and, finally, how to formulate an assessment statement.

TERMINAL OBJECTIVES

MODULE GOAL
The overall goal is to help the student acquire the following knowledges and skills basic to physical health assessment:

1. application of knowledge and understanding of the health history in the physical health assessment process
2. knowledge of the data to be gathered during a physical examination
3. knowledge of and beginning skill development in the following techniques of physical examination: inspection, palpation, percussion, and auscultation
4. knowledge of a systematic way to formulate an assessment statement

The goal is *not* to make the student proficient in doing a complete history and physical examination. Rather, it is to assist her to acquire selected knowledges and skills needed for physical assessment and to help her develop a systematic approach to assessing health status.

OVERALL OBJECTIVES
1. Given questions on selected parts of the physical examination, the student will identify information to be gathered during a physical examination.

© 1977 Wiley

2. Given appropriate questions, models, or examples, the student will identify or describe the proper techniques and the data to be gathered when doing inspection, palpation, percussion, and auscultation.
3. Given a manikin or classmate, the student will demonstrate proper technique and systematic method of palpation, percussion, and auscultation.
4. Given a hypothetical client situation, the student will demonstrate ability to gather data about a specific complaint and develop an assessment statement.

SPECIFIC LEARNING OBJECTIVES
These are located at the beginning of each Activity of this module. They are derived from the overall objectives but specify more precise behaviors that the student will achieve.

Prerequisites

LEARNER PREREQUISITE KNOWLEDGE
1. The normal size, shape, location, and function of the structures in each of the body systems.
2. Knowledge and understanding of common pathophysiological conditions for each body system. Examples: allergic rhinitis, asthma, bronchitis, coronary infarction, urinary tract infections, etc. Further examples of common pathophysiological conditions may be found in Taber's *Encyclopedic Medical Dictionary*.
3. Knowledge and skill related to taking vital signs and using the stethoscope. Knowledge of use of otoscope, ophthalmoscope, and other physical examination instruments is needed, but skill in their use is not essential for this module.
4. Knowledge of and skill in interviewing techniques.
5. Knowledge of data to be gathered in a health history, or completion of the module *The Nursing History*.
6. Knowledge of the process of assessment, or completion of the modules *Psychosocial Assessment* and *Physical Health Assessment*.

Resources Needed

1. ITRAN series *Physical Diagnosis*—five slide-cassette programs including: A Nursing Overview, History Taking, Inspection, Palpation and Percussion, and Auscultation.[1]
2. Sponge block models—directions on how to construct included with activities related to palpation.
3. Stethoscope.
4. Record—"Normal and Abnormal Breath Sounds."[2]

General Learner Tasks

1. Take module Pretest and score it using the Pretest answers.
2. If your Pretest score meets the requirements stated, you need not complete this module.
3. If your Pretest score does not meet all the requirements stated, review the Pretest with your instructor or preceptor, relating the questions to the learning objectives. Decide together

---

[1] Available from ITRAN Training Systems, 1505 Fourth Street, Santa Monica, Calif. 90401.
[2] Available from St. Vincent's Hospital, 153 West 11th Street, New York, N.Y. 10011.

© 1977 Wiley

whether you should complete the entire module or only those learning activities related to the objectives you didn't demonstrate adequately.
4. Proceed to each of the areas decided upon and complete the learning activities as directed.
5. Take the Posttest and score it using the Posttest answers.
6. If your Posttest score meets the requirements stated, you have successfully completed this module.
7. If your Posttest score is below that required, do the following:
    a. Return to the learning activities and do any that you have not previously completed.
    b. Read any of the materials on the Reference List, found at the end of this module, that may be related to the areas you have not yet accomplished.
    c. Retake the Posttest and score it with the answers.
    d. Return both Posttests to your instructor or preceptor and decide together on your next action.
8. Completion of this module should not be attempted in one day. You will need time for content review and for practice with someone else for skill development. It is suggested that the student read the learning objectives, located at the beginning of each Activity, and the learning activities for each Activity and then develop a plan for completion that allows for appropriate breaks and practice time.

ACTIVITY 1
HEALTH HISTORY

The information obtained from the client about his health status is known as the health history. It is a most valuable first step in assessment for several reasons. First, the nurse uses it to develop rapport with the client by getting to know and understand him and his environment. At the same time, the client has an opportunity to "size up" the nurse, doctor, or health team member taking the history. Second, the history is used to elicit valuable diagnostic information. Third, the information obtained through the history provides a focus for the physical examination and gives some insight into the client's functional status, even before examination. Last, information gathered during history taking often points to laboratory studies and therapy to follow.

It is assumed that the student using this module has already completed the module on *Taking a Nursing History* or has previous knowledge of data to be gathered for a health history. Application of this knowledge will be required in Activity 7. Since the health history is such a vital part of the physical assessment, development of the art of history taking is essential, and this requires practice and conscientious efforts to improve.

ACTIVITY 2
PHYSICAL EXAMINATION

The specific learning objectives for this part are the following:

1. Given the steps of a physical examination, the student will
    (a) order them in a logical sequence and
    (b) state rationale for the order.

© 1977 Wiley

2. Given questions on selected parts of the physical examination—for example, the cardiovascular system—the student will identify information to be gathered during the examination.

The physical examination should be an orderly, systematic process employing the four techniques of inspection, palpation, percussion, and auscultation in every body area in order to gather data for the physical assessment. The examining techniques should be carried out as gently as possible. All findings, both normal and abnormal, should be recorded as accurately as possible and in quantitative terms, such as millimeters or cubic centimeters.

The intent of this part of the module is *not* to teach the student to perform a complete physical examination, but rather to help her learn what data are gathered during the physical examination and the four basic techniques for gathering them. Not all states, as yet, have nurse practice acts that sanction an expanded role of the nurse so that prepared nurses can do complete physical examinations. However, the nurse should know and utilize all these examination techniques when assessing any symptoms of which the client has complained or when gathering data for the assessment of any newly admitted client.

Using a systematic format when examining clients helps insure completeness. One suggested format or sequence of steps for a general physical examination of an adult is as follows:

1. Initial vital signs are taken with the client sitting before the examination is started.
2. Examine the head and neck, back, and posterior chest. This starts a head-to-toe order for the examination. The sitting puts the client on a comparable level with the examiner in this early phase when rapport is just getting established, and it allows for comparison of physiological functions, such as blood pressure, once the position of the client is changed.
3. The client should then be asked to lie down, and the blood pressure rechecked. Examination of most of the body parts in this step is facilitated by the recumbent position. The heart, lungs, breasts, axillae, abdomen, genitalia (for males), and extremities are examined. Most of the neurological and orthopedic examinations are also done while the client is recumbent, but certain features, such as analysis of gait, require an upright position.
4. Last, the rectal examination is done for the male or the pelvic-rectal for the female client. By this point there has usually been sufficient opportunity for the establishment of rapport so that optimum client comfort and cooperation can be achieved.

For infants and children the sequence of examination is usually different from that for adults. Investigation of those systems of the body requiring the greatest relaxation and causing the least discomfort, such as auscultation of the chest and palpation of the abdomen, are performed first. Those areas that may cause discomfort, such as the nose, throat, and ears, should be examined last.

The various body parts or systems evaluated during a physical examination and the type of data that should be gathered for each area are as follows:

Vital Statistics: Sex, height, weight, race, age, temperature, pulse rate and rhythm, respiratory rate, blood pressure (right and left arms, sitting and recumbent).

General Physical and Cognitive State: Speech, nutrition, independent ambulation, prostheses, indwelling tubes, striking symptoms such as pallor, cyanosis, constant coughing, respiratory distress, voice abnormality; general behavior, orientation, concentration, abstract thinking, judgment and comprehension, perceptivity, signs of anxiety, cooperation during exam.

Skin: Color, texture, moisture, temperature; amount, texture, and distribution of hair; surgical or traumatic scars. Detailed description of any eruption, abnormal pigmentation, or skin tumor.

Lymph Nodes: Enlargement (recorded in centimeters), consistency, mobility, tenderness.

Head: Size, shape, contour, asymmetry, tenderness over sinuses or mastoids.

Eyes: Protrusion or ptosis, conjunctivae, sclerae, pupillary size and reaction to light and accommodation. Finger is used to test extraocular muscle, gross visual fields, and intraocular

© 1977 Wiley

pressure. Ophthalmoscope is used for evaluation of the optic disc, blood vessels, and macula of the retina.

Ears: Test for hearing acuity: Tuning fork used for Weber's test (to check equal perception of sound in both ears) and Rinne test (for comparison of air and bone conduction). Mastoid process and pinna are inspected. Otoscope used for external canal inspection, looking for foreign bodies, discharge, lesions, edema, inflammation, and the tympanic membrane—color, bulging, inflammation, scars, perforations, and general anatomical appearance.

Nose: Septal deviation, airway obstruction, discharge, condition of mucosa, enlargement of turbinates, polyps. When sinus disease is suspected, transilluminate the sinuses.

Mouth and Throat: Odor of breath; color and appearance of lips, tongue, gums; condition of teeth; dentures; appearance of mucosa, palate, uvula, tonsils, and posterior pharynx. When indicated by symptoms, the nasopharynx and larynx are examined.

Neck: Rigidity or limitation of motion, abnormal pulsation, scars, masses, enlarged salivary glands or lymph nodes; position of trachea and description of thyroid, if palpable.

Back: Contour and mobility of spine; kyphosis, scoliosis, or lordosis. Tenderness on palpation.

Thorax and Lungs: Inspection of thorax for configuration, symmetry, respiratory movements, lesions. Palpation for symmetry of tactile fremitus, masses, and tenderness. Percussion of chest for symmetry of sound, boundaries of thoracic cavity, and excursion of diaphragm. Auscultation for character of breath and voice sounds, and presence of rales, wheezes, rhonchi, or friction rub.

Breasts: Size, consistency, symmetry, tenderness, discharge from nipples, palpable masses.

Cardiovascular: Inspection of the precordium for abnormal pulsations, bulging, or heaving, and for the location of the apical impulse. Systematic palpation of the entire precordium is done for impulses, shocks, thrills, and rubs, noting their location and timing. Percussion is used to define the area of cardiac dullness, and this is measured in centimeters. Systematic ausculation over the entire precordium, especially at valve areas, is done to determine the character of rate, rhythm, quality of sounds, extra sounds, murmurs, and rubs.

Abdomen: Inspection for general appearance, symmetry, hair distribution, scars, local prominences, distention, retraction, dilated blood vessels, pulsations, and any intrinsic movements. Palpation, noting size of liver, spleen, and inguinal nodes; femoral pulses; presence of tenderness, guarding, rigidity, hyperesthesis, fluid, masses, and hernias. Percussion to determine borders of liver, spleen, masses, and the presence of fluid. Auscultation for peristaltic activity and bruits.

Genitalia: (Male) Inspection of penis for lesions and discharge; palpation for tenderness or swelling. Palpation of scrotum for spermatic cords, testes, and epididymis. (Female) Genitalia are examined at the time of the pelvic and rectal exams.

Extremities and Orthopedic Examination: Joints are examined for swelling, tenderness, redness, heat, deformity, and limitation of motion. Nails are checked for clubbing, cyanosis, and abnormality. Peripheral pulses are checked for character, volume, and rate. Extremities are checked for edema, color, temperature, tenderness (especially calf tenderness—Homan's sign), and trophic changes or ulcerations. Musculature is evaluated for size, shape, symmetry, and strength. Characteristics of posture, gait, and movements are observed during the entire encounter with the client.

Neurologic Examination: In a routine physical examination, testing is done of the deep tendon reflexes, pathologic reflexes, proprioceptive sense, and any gross sensory disturbances or muscle weakness. In cases of suspected neurologic disease, this system is examined completely.

Rectum: Inspection for anal pigmentation, thickened skin, excoriation, inflammation, hemorrhoids, and lesions or rashes. Palpation for sphincter tone, masses, tender area, swellings, fissures or fistulas. For males, the size, shape, symmetry and consistency of prostate gland is determined.

© 1977 Wiley

Pelvic Examination (for females): Inspection for normal size, shape, and development of labia majora and minora, clitoris, and urethral and vaginal orifices. Observation for inflammation, ulceration, and discharge; if present, cultures are made. Palpation of the labia, Bartholin and Skene's glands, and perineal musculature is done for masses and tenderness. The vagina, fornices, and cervix are inspected with the aid of the speculum. Size, shape, and coloring of these structures are evaluated, and observation is made for presence of inflammation, ulceration, and discharge (if abnormal discharge is present, culture is made). Papanicolaou smear is done for cytology. Palpation (bimanually) is done to determine size, shape, position, and any irregularities of the cervix, uterus, and ovaries. Rectovaginal examination may be done to access the strength of supporting structures and to evaluate the rectum (as previously described).

There are some differences in the data gathered during the examination of infants and children because of the rapid changes in growth and development. For example, the head and sometimes the chest of an infant or young child is measured in addition to the height and weight. These are usually plotted on a graph and compared to established norms for sex and age. Determination of the rate of growth is especially important during periods of rapid growth, such as infancy and adolescence. Owing to immaturity of the nervous system at birth, the reflex pattern differs from that in the normal adult, with such reflexes as the sucking, rooting, moro, grasp, and tonic neck all being normal at birth but decreasing and disappearing during the first few weeks or months. Some parts of the routine adult physical examination, such as digital examination of the rectum and vagina, are reserved for children with diagnostic problems, intraabdominal complaints, or neurologic disorders. Along with physiological growth, the language, social, intellectual, and emotional development are carefully assessed in cultural context, during the physical examination. Considering any of these out of context culturally could lead to an inaccurate assessment.

The approach used by the examiner during the physical examination varies greatly with the age of the patient. Play techniques are important in gaining cooperation of the young. A very slow, deliberate approach is often important with the elderly.

PROGRESS CHECK

The following are designed to promote mastery of the objectives stated at the beginning of Activity 2.

1. Read any nursing or medical textbook that explains the components of the physical examination. Look for the suggested performance sequence as well as the data to be gathered by examination. Try to rationalize any differences in the textbook information and that given in Activity 2 of this module.

2. Read at least three examples of client history and physical examinations on medical records or in textbooks. Compare the content to the information you have studied in this module and in the textbooks. Select one of the history and physicals reviewed and write down the data gathered in three areas that are particularly significant to the client's chief complaint. List additional information that could have been included in these three areas.

3. Observe a nurse or doctor doing a complete history and physical examination. List the steps she uses when performing the physical examination in the order performed. Critique the completed history and physical examination. You may want to ask about differences in procedure or content from the "textbook picture," recognizing that experienced practitioners are often skilled in individualizing their approach to the patient's needs.

4. Now, review objectives at the beginning of Activity 2 and see if you can perform the actions called for in each. Review the module and textbook material until you are very familiar with the total content.

© 1977 Wiley

ACTIVITY 3
INSPECTION

The specific learning objective for this part is the following: Given a list of the following five areas included in a general inspection, the student will identify three observations to be made for each area by inspection.

a. body features
b. state of consciousness and cognitive state
c. speech
d. body movement
e. outstanding signs

The first fundamental technique used to gather data for the physical examination is inspection. It is the least mechanical but possibly the most difficult of the four techniques because it requires astute observation, which must be cultivated. Many times special tools, such as otoscopes, ophthalmoscopes, or speculae, are used to assist the examiner to visualize a body part during inspection. This module does not teach how to use these instruments, but it does include the data one would be observing for when inspecting with the aid of an instrument. In inspection, it is knowing how to observe and how to interpret what is observed that requires skill.

The following suggestions are designed to help the student master the above objective.

Activities

1. We all need periodic practice with general observational skills. Sharpening observational skills requires conscious effort and exercise.
    a. Talk to a person for ten minutes. During this time observe the person carefully and in detail. Look at general characteristics, such as height, approximate weight, body build, nutritional state, color of eyes, hair, and skin, age and aging characteristics, scars and other identifying features. Look at general appearance and such things as dress, jewelry, hair style, condition of fingernails, posture, and gait. Look for clues about his or her emotional state, such as attitude, mood, and mannerisms. If he or she appears happy, depressed, sad or anxious, what specific observations lead you to that conclusion?
    b. After the ten-minute observational period, *write down your observations*. This is very important for purposes of recall, verification, and self-evaluation. (Keep this description; you will use it again in the Progress Check.
    c. Verify your written observations by looking at the individual again and/or asking him or her to read and critique your observations. Don't forget to explain your reason for scrutinizing.
2. Do *one* of the following two activities. While doing so, look for the data to be gathered by inspection for each of the five areas stated in the objective for Activity 3. List three observations for each of the five areas.
    a. View the ITRAN slide-cassette program entitled "Physical Diagnosis: Inspection." This program introduces the two levels of inspection: general inspection and systems inspection.
    b. Read the section or sections on general and systems inspection in any nursing or medical textbook designed to teach physical examination. Be sure the part on general inspection covers the areas listed in the objective. Depending on the organization of the textbook, you may need to read parts of several chapters to obtain the data related to inspection for each of the body systems.

© 1977 Wiley

72 NURSING ASSESSMENT

PROGRESS CHECK

1. Review the material in this module on the physical examination.
   a. Identify the information that could be obtained by inspection. This has been done for the thorax and abdomen in Activity 2. For every area of the physical examination, write in additional data to be obtained by inspection.
   b. Review the written observations you made in the first activity of this section. Categorize each observation according to where it would fit in the general or systems inspection. Add any additional observations you may recall at this time and categorize them also.
2. Practice doing a complete general and systems inspection on one of your clients, a friend, or even yourself. It may be more difficult to be objective if you practice on yourself, but the object, at this point, is to both increase your observational power and to begin developing a systematic routine for inspection. After completing the examination, record the data you gathered, using the physical examination format.

ACTIVITY 4

PALPATION

The following are specific learning objectives for this part of the module:

1. Given questions related to the correct technique for palpation, the student will identify (a) technique and systematic method of palpation and (b) the data to be gathered while palpating the following body areas and structures: (1) neck, (2) chest, including the lungs and heart, (3) abdomen, including the liver
2. Given a sponge block model containing a mass, the student will palpate the mass and describe it in terms of its location, size, shape, regularity of borders, consistency, mobility, and tenderness.
3. Given a manikin or willing classmate, the student will demonstrate for an instructor or preceptor the proper technique and systematic method of palpation of either the posterior chest or the abdomen.

Palpation enables an examiner to "visualize" a body structure that can't be seen directly. Many normal body organs and structures, as well as abnormal ones, such as masses or tumors, must be palpated to evaluate the location, size, shape, regularity of borders, consistency, mobility, and tenderness. It is also important to palpate for sounds, such as those generated in the heart by a murmur, in the blood vessels by a thrill, or the bronchi by voice sounds. Remember that the fingertips are the most sensitive for fine tactile discrimination, but the palmar aspects of the metacarpophalangeal joints are most sensitive for perceiving vibration.

In general, palpation is a technique which most nurses need to practice, because in many nursing educational programs little emphasis is placed on using touch as a data-gathering tool. The following learning activities are planned to assist the student in gaining skill in palpation.

Activities

1. View Part I of the ITRAN program "Physical Diagnosis: Palpation and Percussion," or, in any nursing or medical textbook designed to teach physical examination, read the section on palpation. List data that should be gathered by palpating the neck, chest, and abdomen.

© 1977 Wiley

2. Learning to palpate means not only getting the fingers accustomed to feeling, but also getting the mind to interpret what is felt and to describe that accurately. For practice in palpating and describing make sponge block models as directed here and do the following exercises.
    a. Obtain (or cut from a larger piece of foam rubber) three or four foam rubber cubes approximately 3 to 4 inches on each side.
    b. Cut the cubes in half; inside each place one of several small objects of varying size, shape, and consistency; tape or spot-glue the halves together again. The following are suggested objects to use inside the cubes: regular marble, larger "shooter" marble, a small rubber or plastic ball, a grape, a raisin, a prune—cooked or dried, a small piece of styrofoam packing material, an inch-long piece of finger cot that has been filled with water or lubricating gel and tied with thread, a piece of twig or bark, a walnut or almond, a pencil eraser.
    c. Practice palpating the objects in the cubes, one at a time. First, practice just holding the cube between your hands. This is similar to palpating a mass directly between two layers of body tissue. Next, practice palpating the mass with the cube placed on a solid surface, such as a table top, and then on a soft surface, such as a pillow. Remember, in the body some masses develop over solid areas such as bones or ribs and other masses develop in "softer" areas such as the abdomen. When palpating, notice the difference in the "feel" of the object when the underlying structure has a different consistency.
    d. Ask somebody else to change the object in one cube and to place it on a table. Now, palpate the cube without removing it from the table, and write a description of the "mass" in the cube. Include the following in your description.
        1. Location—You may use any division scheme on the cube, such as quadrants, points on the face of a clock, etc., or you may use the borders of the cube as points of reference and measure the distance from these to locate the mass. Don't forget such terms as anterior, posterior, medial, and lateral.
        2. Size—Estimate this in centimeters; try to include length, width, and depth when appropriate.
        3. Shape—Use geometric figures or some common object, such as a walnut or egg, to help describe the shape.
        4. Consistency—Use the resistance of the mass to pressure or its firmness to help evaluate this. Is it stony-hard, soft, spongy, or gelatinous?
        5. Regularity of the borders—Decide how the surface of the mass feels. Is it smooth, nodular, regular or irregular, or possibly grooved?
        6. Mobility—How does the mass respond to direct attempts to displace it? Is it freely mobile? Does it move in response to the movement of an adjacent structure? (This indicates attachment to that structure.)
        7. Tenderness—Of course, your sponge model will not complain of tenderness, but if you were examining a person, you would record any tenderness or pain associated with a mass.
        8. Any other distinguishing characteristics—Occasionally you may notice some other characteristics when examining a mass, and these must also be recorded. An example is the pulsatility of an aneurysm.
        After writing your description, open the cube and compare your description with the actual "mass" to see how accurately you palpated and described the object in the cube.
3. Now, practice palpating and describing a couple of normal anatomical structures on yourself or a friend. The following are some suggested structures for your palpating practice: the patella, a small bone in a finger or toe, the submaxillary salivary gland. Check your description of the structure palpated against that given in an anatomy book.

PROGRESS CHECK

1. Review palpation of the chest in the ITRAN program or your reading. On a friend or client practice a systematic method of palpating the posterior chest, including evalua-

tion of respiratory expansion and vocal fremitus. Remember the following key points:
   a. Use both hands simultaneously and palpate symmetrical areas of the thorax from above down during normal and deep respiration.
   b. To test vocal fremitus ask the person to repeat a resonant phrase, such as "ninety-nine," while palpating all lung segments from above down.
   c. Evaluate the degree and symmetry of expansion with respiration, and evaluate comparative increase, decrease or absence of vocal fremitus.
2. Review the part of your reading or the ITRAN program related to palpation of the abdomen, then do the following two activities. The main objectives for this practice should be (1) to determine what a normal abdomen "feels" like, and (2) to decide on some systematic approach to palpating the abdomen that seems comfortable and logical to you.
   a. Practice light and deep palpation on yourself or someone else, trying out a couple of different systematic approaches. Remember, in light palpation identify areas that might be normally tender and with deep palpation identify all normal organs and structures that can be palpated.
   b. On a friend or client try to palpate the costal border of the liver in the manner described in the ITRAN program or your reading. Write down your findings, and compare these to the norms stated in the reference you are using.

ACTIVITY 5
PERCUSSION

The following are learning objectives for Activity 5:

1. Given a list of body structures with varying degrees of density, the student will describe the normal sounds elicited by percussion.
2. Given examples of data gathered by percussion of the chest and abdomen, the student will describe the significance of the data.
3. Given a manikin or willing classmate, the student will demonstrate for an instructor or preceptor the proper technique and systematic method of bimanual percussion of the posterior chest or the abdomen.

The technique of percussion can be used on any body part but is primarily used in evaluating the chest and abdomen. This technique involves setting the chest or abdominal wall in motion by striking it directly or indirectly and evaluating the sound produced, which is reflective of the structure of the underlying thoracic or abdominal contents. One must become familiar with the range of normal tones produced by percussion. The tone is influenced by the thickness of the wall as well as the density of the underlying structures.

Percussion can be used in the following ways: (1) to assess such normal anatomy as diaphragmatic excursion, the degree to which the diaphragm descends during inspiration and expiration; (2) to map borders of underlying structures and thus determine the size of those structures (or levels, in the case of fluid); (3) to determine the density of underlying structures and assess normalcy or confirm the abnormal presence of fluid, masses, or consolidation. An example of the latter is the percussion of lung tissue to assess density. Increased resonance of the lung upon percussion indicates overinflation of the tissue or emphysema, whereas decreased resonance is indicative of fluid or pleural thickening.

The following activities are designed to help nursing students develop beginning skill in performing percussion and in evaluating the data gained.

© 1977 Wiley

Activities

1. View Part II of the ITRAN program entitled "Physical Diagnosis: Palpation and Percussion" or read in any nursing or medical text designed to teach the technique and significance of percussion. Study particularly the content related to the knowledge and skills called for in the objectives for this Activity.

2. Make a list of the following body parts or areas: head (skull), forearm, upper arm, chest over lung after deep inspiration, chest over lung after expiration, chest over heart, stomach, liver, abdomen on each side of the umbilicus, thigh. Think about the density of each part, and write down the sound (tympany, hyperresonance, resonance, dull, flat) you would anticipate hearing if you were to percuss that body part. Now, perform the technique of percussion over each body part/area and write down the sound you hear. Compare the two lists of answers. Do the answers match?

3. When you were percussing the area around the umbilicus on the abdomen, the sound elicited was tympany or hyperresonance. What might be the significance of hearing dullness in this area upon percussion? (Answer: If you suspect fluid or a mass in the abdominal cavity, you are beginning to understand the importance of percussion to physical assessment.)

4. As you have learned, percussion is also used to map the borders of organs and thus determine their size. Practice percussion of the liver on a friend or client. Remember the following key points:
   a. Percuss down on the right side in the midclavicular line to the upper border of the liver (level of dullness), usually at the 6th intercostal space. Don't forget that a wedge of lung intervenes between the liver and chest wall at this point so that the transition from lung resonance to hepatic dullness may be subtle. Listen carefully: A review of illustrations in your textbook or in the ITRAN program will be helpful.
   b. Percuss up on the right side in the midclavicular line to the lower border, usually at the costal margin.
   c. Measure the distance between the upper and lower borders in the midclavicular line. Normal size is usually about 10 cm; normal range is from 8 cm in a small person to 12 cm in a large man.

PROGRESS CHECK

On a friend or client practice percussion of the posterior chest and the abdomen, as described in the ITRAN program or your reading. The following are some key points to remember:

a. The technique employs the middle finger of the left hand to press against the skin, with the other fingers on that hand not touching the skin. The middle finger of the right hand strikes the base of the distal phalanx of the finger pressed against the skin. The striking motion is a wrist action, the blow being sharp and quick. (This is the indirect percussion technique.)

b. Percussion should be done systematically. On the posterior chest it should be from side to side sequentially from the suprascapular area downward to the lung base. The middle finger pressed firmly against the chest wall should be in the intercostal spaces and parallel to the ribs. On the abdomen, percussion (and palpation) should follow auscultation and should be done in some chosen pattern that includes all areas of the abdomen.

c. Tone quality and changes of tone quality should be identified to determine the borders and density of underlying structures.

d. Write down your findings after performing percussion of the posterior chest and the abdomen. Compare these to the norms given in your reference.

© 1977 Wiley

ACTIVITY 6
AUSCULTATION

The learning objectives for this Activity are the following:

1. The student will demonstrate knowledge of the following by correctly answering all objective questions on auscultation.
    a. the difference between the bell and diaphragm headpieces of the stethoscope,
    b. the *specific* areas of the neck, chest, and abdomen for which auscultation is used and the normal sounds that would be expected in these areas,
    c. a definition and description of the following abnormal sounds: bruits, asthmatic breath sounds, rales, pleural friction rub, gallop rhythm, tic-tac rhythm, murmur, and peritoneal fiction rub,
    d. the three types of information to listen for during auscultation of the various areas of the heart.
2. Given a manikin or classmate, the student will demonstrate for an instructor or preceptor correct auscultation, including technique and systematic method, of *two* of the following:
    a. the chest for heart sounds
    b. the chest for breath sounds (include both anterior and posterior chest)
    c. the abdomen

Sound within the body is produced primarily in one of two ways: by the movement of air through hollow structures or by the forces that move columns of fluid and set solid structures in motion. Some of the body sounds of clinical importance are breath sounds (the movement of air through the trachea and bronchi), voice sounds (air moving past functioning vocal cords), bowel sounds (air moving through the intestines), heart sounds (the impedance to flowing blood caused by closed valves and the heart wall), and murmurs (the moving of blood through vascular structures that cause resistance to flow). Sometimes normal sounds are distorted by pathology of structures through which the sound must travel. For example, the character of breath sounds change when they must travel through the consolidated lung of lobar pneumonia. Therefore, the ability to recognize normal body sounds and to understand the significance of changed sounds is a very important aspect in the physical examination and in the total physical health assessment, which is done when all the data are compiled.

The following learning activities are planned to help the student develop beginning skill in auscultation and the recognition of normal physiological sounds. When working on these activities, refer frequently to the Learning Objectives.

Activities

1. View the ITRAN program "Physical Diagnosis: Auscultation," or read in any nursing or medical textbook, designed to teach physical assessment, the parts related to the use of the stethoscope and the technique of auscultation. Remember to identify and study the knowledges called for in the objectives, Activity 6, such as definitions, etc.
2. Practice identifying breath sounds:
    a. After reviewing the description and location of the three types of normal breath sounds in your reading or the ITRAN program, try locating and listening to these on a healthy person. Listen on both the anterior and the posterior chest with the objectives of (1) identifying the three types of normal breath sounds and (2) identifying their normal location. Listen with both the bell and the diaphragm stethoscope chestpieces and make your own comparisons. Do *you* hear breath sounds more clearly with the bell or diaphragm?

© 1977 Wiley

b. Next listen to normal voice sounds with the stethoscope. Have your healthy "client" whisper repeatedly a resonant phrase, such as "ninety-nine," and listen over the entire chest for the sound and changes in the sound. Where are the voice sounds loudest? softest? What do you think causes the change in intensity? What might cause the voice sounds to have an increased intensity? a diminished intensity?

   Did you decide that conditions that interpose something between the lung and chest wall, such as fluid (pleural effusion) or air (pneumothorax), decrease voice sound intensity, whereas a condition, such as consolidation, that improves sound transmission increases the voice sounds?

c. Listen to the recording "Normal and Abnormal Breath Sounds." Try to become familiar with some of the abnormal breath sounds and adventitious sounds, such as moist and dry rales and friction rubs. If at all possible, listen to the breath sounds of any client with respiratory difficulties. Try to identify the sounds you hear and verify your decisions with an instructor or preceptor.

4. Practice identifying heart sounds.
   a. Review the ITRAN program or your reading to refresh your memory on the cardiac cycle, auscultatory valve areas, and heart sounds.
   b. Listen to your own heart and do the following:
      (1) Locate all four auscultatory valve areas.
      (2) Listen to the sounds in each area using this order: aortic, pulmonic, mitral, and tricuspid. Use the bell; then repeat the pattern using the diaphragm.
      (3) Determine where the first sound is loudest; then determine where the second is loudest.
   c. Using the same systematic pattern, listen to the heart sounds of another healthy person. Compare the heart sounds of the other person to your own.
   d. If at all possible, listen to the heart sounds of a person with known cardiac pathology. Compare and contrast those heart sounds to the normal ones you heard and verify your comparison with an instructor or preceptor.

5. Practice listening to abdominal sounds.
   a. On yourself or another healthy person, practice auscultation of the abdomen.
   b. Use the same systematic pattern for auscultation of the abdomen that you developed when practicing inspection, palpation, and percussion. Remember, however, that if you were actually examining a client, auscultation would follow inspection and precede palpation or percussion.
   c. With the stethoscope, using the diaphragm, listen in all areas of the abdomen for peristaltic and vascular sounds. Write down your findings and compare them to the norms given in your references.

ACTIVITY 7

DEVELOPING A STATEMENT OF PHYSICAL HEALTH ASSESSMENT

The following is the learning objective for this final Activity: Given an example of a complaint involving the respiratory system, the student will describe a systematic approach to assessing this system, including the following in his description:

a. initial observations to be made by general inspection

b. information to be obtained about the present illness when taking the health history

© 1977 Wiley

78 NURSING ASSESSMENT

    c. data gathered by each of the four techniques (inspection, palpation, percussion, auscultation)
    d. how to use the data to formulate an assessment statement

Now that you have learned about the health history and physical examination and have developed some beginning skills in the four basic examination techniques, you need to be able to put these all together for use with clients and to communicate to others the data obtained in a logical concise manner. That is the goal of this final Activity.

The assessment statement reflects the similarities and differences between the data gathered from the client and the usual progression or development patterns in health and disease. The statement is developed in the following way: (1) reviewing and tabulating all the data obtained from the history, physical examination, and laboratory tests; (2) eliminating irrelevant material and condensing relevant findings; (3) comparing the tabulated data with a known body of knowledge, such as that obtained from textbooks, experts, and experience; and (4) writing a statement or statements that reflect the degree of correspondence between the client's findings and the known patterns of health and disease. The following learning activity will assist you in "putting it all together" and developing an assessment statement.

Activity

In this module's final Activity you are given a brief hypothetical client situation with step-by-step directions and questions to help you to assess the client's physical complaints. Role-play the hypothetical situation and your physical assessment with a classmate or friend who will consent to your examination. Write answers to the activity questions and develop your assessment statement. Then compare your actions, thoughts, and assessment statement to the answers given.

HYPOTHETICAL CASE
Lynn Jensen, a 26-year-old married college student at U.C.L.A., comes to you with the complaint of nasal discharge and cough of one week's duration.

1. As the client describes the complaints to you initially, you should make a rapid but careful general inspection. What are some of the specific observations you would make?

2. Interview the client to gather specific data about the complaint. In other words, take a health history. In this activity you need only write down data about the present illness. What are four points in the history of the present illness about which you should gather information? What data should you elicit about each point? Write your observations and history of the present illness.

© 1977 Wiley

3. Examine your client to gather physical signs, especially related to the thorax and lungs. Use all four examination techniques and record your findings. What kind of data will you gather during inspection? palpation? percussion? auscultation? (You may want to write down the answer to this question before conducting your examination.)

4. Obtain data from routine and specialized laboratory tests, such as X-rays, blood tests, respiratory function tests, etc. (Laboratory tests were not included as part of this module, but in this hypothetical case one would expect to evaluate results of chest X-ray, looking for any cause of bronchial constriction or obstruction; nasal smear and blood tests for eosinophils; and skin tests for allergens, such as tree pollens.)

5. The next step in formulating an assessment statement is to tabulate all data and construct a logical report or record, eliminating irrelevant material and condensing relevant findings. For the purposes of this exercise, go back over your written history of the present illness and physical examination report and underline the data you would include in this summary. Include only the most pertinent parts of the history and only the positive physical findings (such as wheezing, in this case).

6. Compare your summarized, tabulated data with a known body of knowledge, such as obtained from textbooks, experts, and experience. What kind of knowledge do you need in order to evaluate this client's symptoms, and where will you find it? Write a brief comparison of the client's symptoms and the data you found during your research.

80 NURSING ASSESSMENT

7. The last step is to write a statement that reflects the degree of correspondence between your findings and known patterns of health and disease. Now, write your assessment of Lynn's chief complaint.

ANSWERS

1. The general inspection should include observations related to body features, state of consciousness, speech, body movement, and outstanding signs, especially those associated with and verifying the client's complaints, such as coughing, nasal dripping, dyspnea, cyanosis, wheezing or sneezing.

2. When gathering information about the present illness, obtain: (a) an elaboration of the chief complaint that includes symptom characteristics, character of the complaint, location, intensity or severity, timing, aggravating and relieving factors, and associated symptoms; (b) a history of the present problem that includes data on manner of onset and precipitating and predisposing factors related to onset; (c) a description of the present status of the problem including the course since onset, incidence or occurrences of symptoms, progress and effect of any therapy; (d) a summary of all significant positives and negatives related to the symptoms that have been elicited from a review of systems, or in this case at least a review of the respiratory system.

Sample history: Lynn Jensen, a 26-year-old (male or female depending on your role-playing partner), married college student at U.C.L.A., comes with a chief complaint of nasal discharge and cough of one week's duration. Client appears well nourished with no obvious scars or deformities and in no acute distress, although does cough and wipe nose occasionally. Patient says the rhinorrhea is accompanied by sneezing and itchy eyes, primarily when outside. The cough, which is dry, tight, and paroxysmal, began about the same time as the clear, watery nasal discharge. Coughing occasionally leads to expectoration of small amount of thick, white sputum. Client states she has also experienced dyspnea after mild exertion, such as walking rapidly to class, and notices an increase in symptoms when outside. For the past three days headaches in the supraorbital region have accompanied other symptoms.

Client states she usually does get "a cold" every spring, but the symptoms this year seem much worse since moving near father-in-law's citrus grove, where Lynn works part-time.

Since onset the rhinorrhea and paroxysmal cough have been continual, the dyspnea has increased, with less exertion causing difficult breathing and coughing, and intermittent headaches have accompanied other symptoms during last three days. Headaches are relieved by aspirin, and client states a nonprescription decongestant drug, taken once a day for past three days, has helped relieve the rhinorrhea. Cough and dyspnea also decrease once rhinorrhea is relieved.

There have been no fever, chest pain, palpitations, cyanosis, night sweats, or edema. Client is not sure about occurrence of wheezing, although she says that on occasion, when dyspneic, breathing has been "rough." Does not know of any allergies, but says father has been diagnosed as having bronchial asthma.

© 1977 Wiley

3. *Inspection* of the chest should include evaluation of its configuration, symmetry, and character of respiratory movements and observation of skin color, pigmentation, scars, and lesions. During *palpation* the following should be evaluated: temperature, texture and moisture of skin, fremitus, extent and symmetry of respiratory expansion, masses, and tenderness. *Percussion* of the chest should include evaluation of the symmetry of sound, abnormal sounds, boundaries of the thoracic cavity and diaphragmatic excursion. *Auscultation* should be done to evaluate the character of breath and voice sounds and to determine the presence of rales, wheezes, rhonchi, or friction rubs.

   Sample record of chest examination: The thorax is symmetrical and of normal configuration with equal expansion during respiration. Position of the diaphragm is normal, and diaphragmatic excursion is 5 centimeters. Fremitus, breath, and voice sounds are normal, but occasional expiratory wheezes are present.

4 & 5. No answer needed.

6. You need data on allergic conditions and conditions characterized by wheezing, such as asthma. Such information can be found in various nursing textbooks, books on pathology, or medical handbooks.

   Sample summarized comparison of client symptoms and textbook data (in reality, this is a mental process and is not ordinarily written on the client's record in this manner): Lynn Jensen's signs and symptoms of rhinorrhea with watery discharge, sneezing, itchy eyes, and frontal headache are the same as those associated with allergic rhinitis. The onset of the client's symptoms being early spring and the worsening of the symptoms on exposure to a citrus grove are factors suggestive of allergy to citrus tree pollen. The client's mild dyspnea, the tight paroxysmal cough which occasionally produces thick, white sputum, the wheezing heard on auscultation, and the family history of bronchial asthma are all factors associated with the textbook picture of bronchial asthma.

7. *Sample assessment statement:* Lynn Jensen is a 26-year-old, well-developed (male/female) college student in no acute distress, having symptoms of allergic rhinitis, possibly due to citrus tree pollen. There is a family history of bronchial asthma, and client is developing signs of this also. (If your assessment statement is similar to this, you are ready to proceed to the module Posttest!)

POSTTEST

The Posttest is divided into two parts. Part A is a mixture of objective and discussion questions. The student can evaluate and score these questions using the Posttest answers. Part B has demonstration questions, which must be performed for an instructor or preceptor.

Part A Circle the *letter* indicating the correct answer on all multiple-choice questions. Answer all other questions as directed. Each question is worth 1 point unless otherwise indicated.

1. The following are the steps in one logical format for a physical examination. State a rationale for the order of each step. (6 points)

   Steps

   1. vital signs, head, neck, back, posterior chest

   Rationale

   1.

82 NURSING ASSESSMENT

    2. blood pressure, heart, lungs, breasts, axillae, abdomen, genitalia, extremities   2.

    3. rectal or pelvic and rectal examinations   3.

2. Match the description of data to be gathered with the body part or system being examined. (6 points)

Data	Body Part or System
____ surgical or traumatic scars	a. abdomen
____ tenderness over sinuses	b. skin
____ evaluation of disc, blood vessels, macula	c. neurological
____ results of Rinne test	d. cardiovascular
____ character of femoral pulses	e. eye
____ evaluation of deep tendon reflexes	f. ear
	g. head
	h. extremities and orthopedic

3. List three general body features for which the nurse would observe when doing a general inspection. (6 points)

4. Which of the following are descriptive of systematic palpation of the abdomen? Indicate the letter that gives the correct combination of responses.
   1. Palpation is done from the suprapubic area to the epigastrium and from the umbilical area to each flank.
   2. The client is placed in recumbent position with the legs extended.
   3. The examiner begins palpating in the area where the patient has complained of tenderness or discomfort.
   4. When palpating the liver, clients should be asked to hold their breath momentarily.
      a. 1 only
      b. 1, 2, 3
      c. 1, 2, 4
      d. all of these

5. List three structures in the neck one would evaluate by palpation. (3 points)

6. List five characteristics of a palpable mass that should be described. (5 points)

7. Write the word describing the normal sound that would be elicited by percussion of each of the body areas listed below. (5 points)
   _____ upper arm
   _____ spleen
   _____ normal lung
   _____ gas-filled bowel
   _____ lung, on deep inspiration

© 1977 Wiley

PHYSICAL HEALTH ASSESSMENT **83**

8. Increased resonance over the lung upon percussion is indicative of (a) _____. Decreased resonance is indicative of (b) _____. (2 points)

9. If the bell headpiece on the stethoscope is held too tightly against the body, the skin is stretched. Why is this undesirable?
   a. It causes the client discomfort.
   b. It causes all sounds to be obliterated.
   c. It causes the closing off of low-pitched sounds.
   d. It causes the closing off of high-pitched sounds.

10. _____ are abnormal swishing sounds, synchronous with the pulse, which might be heard over the carotid arteries when listening with a stethoscope.

11. Match the type of breath sound with its location. (3 points)
    ___ bronchial   a. heard over most normal lung tissue
    ___ bronchovesicular   b. heard normally only over the trachea
    ___ vesicular   c. heard when lung tissue overlies the large bronchi

12. The following statements relate to auscultation of the heart. Write *T* if the statement is true and *F* if it is false. (4 points)
    ___ The auscultatory valve areas do not correspond to the anatomic location of the valves themselves.
    ___ The second heart sound is more prominent at the base of the heart.
    ___ The first heart sound is louder than the second sound at the apex.
    ___ The pulmonic auscultatory area is at the second right interspace at the sternal border.

13. Which of the following may be heard when auscultating the abdomen?
    a. Peristalsis
    b. Succession splashes
    c. Vascular sounds
    d. Friction rubs
    e. All of these

14. Mrs. Martin comes to you with a complaint of four days duration: pain in the chest upon deep breathing. Describe how you would assess this respiratory complaint, including the following in your description:
    a. initial observations to be made by a general inspection while listening to the client describe the chief complaint

    b. information to be obtained about the present illness from the history

© 1977 Wiley

84 NURSING ASSESSMENT

　　c.　data related to examination of the thorax and lungs to be gathered when using each of the four techniques: inspection, palpation, percussion, auscultation

　　d.　how to use the data to formulate an assessment statement (12 points—3 for each part)

Part B　The following must be performed for and evaluated by an instructor or preceptor using the guidelines for evaluation in the Posttest answers. The student will demonstrate the skills called for in the objectives on palpation, percussion, and auscultation.

15. You are given a sponge block model containing a mass. Palpate the mass and write a description of it, as you would if you were describing an anatomical mass. (5 points)
16. Using a manikin or classmate, demonstrate for your instructor or preceptor the proper technique for palpation and percussion of the abdomen. Include the following in your demonstration:
    a. systematic method of light palpation to determine tenderness (4 points)
    b. systematic method of deep palpation to determine specific organs, masses, and tenderness (4 points)
    c. percussion of abdomen to determine borders of the liver (4 points)
17. Using a manikin or classmate, demonstrate for your instructor correct auscultation of any *two* of the following:
    a. the anterior chest for heart sounds
    b. the anterior and posterior chest for breath sounds
    c. the abdomen (6 points—3 for each part demonstrated)

Answers

1. (1) In the first step the client is sitting up, thus allowing for easy access to these body parts and for comparison of physiological functioning once the position is changed.
   (2) Examination and evaluation of all the body parts in this step is facilitated by the client's recumbent position.
   (3) The timing of this step has allowed sufficient time for rapport to be established and client cooperation gained.
2. b, g, e, f, a, c

© 1977 Wiley

3. a. position or attitude
   b. state of hydration
   c. gross deformities
4. a
5. Any three of the following: salivary glands, lymph nodes, carotid and subclavian pulses, trachea, thyroid gland, sternomastoid muscle, any masses present
6. Any five of the following: location, size, shape, consistency, regularity of borders, mobility and tenderness.
7. flatness, dullness, resonance, tympany, hyperresonance
8. (a) emphysema or overinflated lung tissue
   (b) fluid or pleural thickening
9. c.
10. Bruits
11. b, c, a
12. *T, T, T, F*
13. e
14. The same answer guidelines may be used for this situational question as those given for Pretest question 15, because both situations require assessment of a complaint involving the respiratory system.

Part B

15. The description of the "mass" must include at least five of the following types of data: location, size, shape, consistency, regularity of borders, mobility, and tenderness.
16. Evaluation guidelines for demonstration of palpation and percussion of the abdomen:
    a. light palpation (must include steps 1, 2, 4, and 6 in demonstration):
       1. Ask client to lie down with knees flexed slightly; helps client relax by breathing through mouth or other relaxing technique; warms hands.
       2. Use flat of hand, not fingertips, pressing only to depth of 1 cm.
       3. Lift hand from skin when changing position.
       4. Consistently use a systematic progression, such as starting in one quadrant and proceeding in a clockwise manner until all four quadrants are examined.
       5. Move slowly.
       6. Identify tender areas.
    b. deep palpation (must include steps 1, 3, 4, 5):
       1. Help client relax using some technique, such as asking client to breathe through mouth.
       2. Use both hands; passive hand against abdominal wall and active hand applying pressure to passive hand.
       3. Use palmar surfaces of fingers for palpation.
       4. Apply pressure slowly, gently, deliberately, and to a depth of 4 cm.
       5. Identify and palpates tender areas last, but generally follows same systematic progression as for light palpation.
    c. percussion (must include all of the following):
       1. Know that the tone produced by percussion over the liver is dull.
       2. Percuss down on the right side in the mid-clavicular line to the upper border of the liver, usually at the 6th or 7th rib.
       3. Percuss up on the right side in the mid-clavicular line to the lower border, usually at the costal margin.
       4. Measure distance between the upper and lower border in the mid-clavicular line. Know that normal size is about 10 cm.

© 1977 Wiley

17. Evaluation guidelines for heart sounds, breath sounds, and abdomen—auscultation demonstration:
    1. heart sounds (must include b, c, and d in demonstration):
        a. Ask client to hold breath while listens.
        b. Start with bell.
        c. Leave chestpiece at each auscultatory valve site for 3–4 seconds, listening in this order: (1) aortic area, (2) pulmonic area, (3) apex or mitral area, (4) tricuspid area.
        d. Repeat pattern using the diaphragm.
    2. breath sounds on posterior and anterior chest (must include c, d, e):
        a. Have client seated.
        b. Tell client to breathe deeply through mouth; demonstrate this.
        c. Use diaphragm headpiece on stethoscope.
        d. Begin on posterior chest at base of lungs and works across upward, comparing symmetrical areas on both sides until reaching apex of lungs. Use this pattern:
        e. Repeat same on anterior chest using similar pattern.
    3. abdomen (must include all three):
        a. Know to auscultate before palpation or percussion.
        b. Use diaphragm.
        c. Listen in all four quadrants and is consistent in using a systematic pattern.

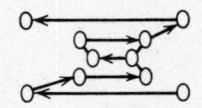

EVALUATION OF ANSWERS FOR SCORING

Part A: Total of 56 points is possible on Part A of the Posttest. A total of *44* points must be correct; in addition, answers to questions 9–13 must be correct to meet criteria stated in the objectives.

Part B: Total of 15 points is possible for the demonstrations; *all* of these points must be earned.

References and Suggested Readings

Brunner, Lillian S., and Suddarth, Doris S., *Textbook of Medical-Surgical Nursing,* 3rd ed. Philadelphia: J. B. Lippincott, 1975.

DeGowin, Elmer L., and DeGowin, Richard L., *Bedside Diagnostic Examination,* 2nd ed. New York: Macmillan, 1969.

Fowkes, William C., and Humm, Virginia K., *Clinical Assessment for the Nurse Practitioner.* St. Louis: C. V. Mosby, 1973.

Judge, Richard D., and Zuidema, George D., *Physical Diagnosis: A Physiologic Approach to the Clinical Examination,* 2nd. ed. Boston: Little, Brown, 1963.

Lehmann, Sister Janet, "Auscultation of heart sounds," *American Journal of Nursing* 72 (1972): 1242–1246.

Littmann, David, "Stethoscopes and auscultation," *American Journal of Nursing* 72 (1972): 1239–1241.

MacBryde, Cyril M., and Blacklow, Robert S., *Signs and Symptoms,* 5th ed. Philadelphia: J. B. Lippincott, 1970.

"Patient assessment: Taking a patient's history," *American Journal of Nursing* 74 (1974): 293–324. Programmed instruction.

Prior, John A., and Silberstein, Jack S., *Physical Diagnosis: The History and Examination of the Patient,* 4th ed. St. Louis: C. V. Mosby, 1973.

© 1977 Wiley

RALPH MATTEOLI, R.N., M.S. (PART 1)
ROBINETTA WHEELER, R.N., M.S. (PART 2)

WILEY NURSING CONCEPT MODULE

PSYCHOSOCIAL ASSESSMENT

CONTENTS

PRETEST 89   Answers 92

PART 1. Stress and Strain 94

INTRODUCTION 94

TERMINAL OBJECTIVES 94

   ACTIVITY 1. Assessment of Stress and Strain 95
   ACTIVITY 2. Assessment of Coping 98
   ACTIVITY 3. Assessment of the Support System 100

PART 2. Arenas of Stress 102

INTRODUCTION 102

TERMINAL OBJECTIVES 103

   ACTIVITY 1. A Framework for Assessing an Arena 103
   ACTIVITY 2. Arena Assessment 105

POSTTEST 113   Answers 117

REFERENCES 118

© 1977 Wiley

PRETEST

PART 1

Directions: Read each statement and circle *T* for True, *F* for False, or the appropriate phrases. When you are done, turn to the answers and correct your own test.

1. A supportive psychosocial environment generally produces positive effects on a client, enhancing growth and development and reducing recovery time from illness. *T F*
2. Stress always produces strain. *T F*
3. Coping means attempting to reduce stress and strain. *T F*
4. The effects of strain are (circle all that apply):
    a. decreased ability to concentrate
    b. unpleasant affective state
    c. disorganization
    d. insomnia
    e. anorexia
    f. tension
    g. decreased coping reserve
5. Changes and losses are stress stimuli that usually produce some degree of strain. *T F*
6. Stresses can accumulate to produce strain. *T F*
7. Changes in one's life can evoke faulty adaptive efforts that can lower bodily resistance to disease. *T F*
8. Productive coping is dealing with reality in a problem-solving way. *T F*
9. Productive coping leads to a stronger sense of self. *T F*
10. Nonproductive coping focuses efforts on decreasing strain alone and the stress goes unresolved. *T F*
11. An active support system helps a client to deal with stress. *T F*
12. The following are behaviors of productive coping (circle all that apply):
    a. clarifies perceptions
    b. seeks information
    c. talks about feelings
    d. uses a variety of defense mechanisms
    e. plans a course of action
    f. executes the plan of action
13. Behaviors that indicate nonproductive coping are (circle all that apply):
    a. uses defense mechanisms
    b. denies or distorts reality
    c. tests reality
    d. uses logical thinking
    e. assumes control over daily life events
    f. is unwilling to participate fully in the experience
    g. is outgoing and seeks others
14. People interacting with the client in a meaningful way make up the support system. *T F*
15. People at work can often be the active support system that the client needs. *T F*
16. A psychosocial environment that is warm and supportive promotes smooth physiological processes. *T F*
17. Behaviors that indicate an active support system are (circle all that apply):
    a. information is freely communicated to the client
    b. expression of feelings is facilitated by the system

© 1977 Wiley

c. all decisions are taken over by the system, thus relieving the client
d. the client's active involvement in the experience is supported

PART 2

1. Match the items on the right with the examples of them in the left column.

   ____1. growth and development providing
   ____2. values
   ____3. innovation
   ____4. mores
   ____5. life, dignity, and integrity promoting
   ____6. family
   ____7. purpose
   ____8. positive change promoting
   ____9. belief system
   ____10. community
   ____11. symbols
   ____12. business
   ____13. organization

   a. culture
   b. arena
   c. process components
   d. purposes of process

2. Write a statement explaining the need for arena assessment.

3. You are applying for a job in the community outreach department of a university medical center. While waiting to be interviewed, you pick up a pamphlet entitled, "Welcome to the Staff of University Medical Center," and read the following:

   "University medical center is an equal opportunity employer. It combines the benefits of an educational facility and a medical center in close proximity. In addition it seeks employees who are interested in a challenge and in continued education. An overview of the unique benefits afforded employees are:

   a. Payment of one-fourth of tuition at University colleges after six months of employment. Increase to one-half payment after one year of employment.
   b. Health and life insurance with a disability insurance option. Health and life insurance are available immediately. Disability insurance is available after six months of employment.
   c. Retirement plan in which the employer contributes one-half, matching the amount contributed by the employee. In the event you leave our employment, the entire amount in your retirement fund will be given to you.
   d. Each employee earns one day per month of sick leave and two days per month of annual leave. Both sick and annual may be used immediately. In special instances, sick leave may be advanced.

   In addition, employees can expect to be considered for promotion every two years automatically. An employee may apply for another position whenever openings are available. Employees will be informed of matters affecting their work through the University Medical Center newspaper and through their supervisors. The University Medical Center conducts in-service presentation per month."

   Sort and list the above information about the University Medical Center into the following five categories, and write an assessment statement.

© 1977 Wiley

Life Dignity, and Integrity Promoting: *Positive Change Promoting:*

Organizational Patterns: *Acquiring and Using New Input:*

Growth and Development Promoting:

Assessment statement:

4. Visit a local health-care agency. Make an assessment of the agency.

5. Below are listed five criteria questions for arena assessment. For each one generate at least five ways in which a community could meet the criteria.
   a. How does the community promote life, dignity, and integrity?

© 1977 Wiley

92 NURSING ASSESSMENT

b. How does the community promote positive change?

c. How does the community promote growth and development?

d. What are the organizational patterns of the community?

e. How does the community acquire and use new information?

Answers

Part 1
1. T
2. F
3. T
4. circle all
5. T
6. T
7. T
8. T
9. T
10. T
11. T
12. circle all except d
13. circle a, b, f, g
14. T
15. T
16. T
17. circle a, b, d

Part 2
1.
  - d 1.
  - a 2.
  - c 3.
  - a 4.
  - d 5.
  - b 6.
  - c 7.
  - d 8.
  - a 9.
  - b 10.
  - a 11.
  - b 12.
  - c 13.

© 1977 Wiley

2. Since the individual is an open system continually interacting with his environment and since arenas are areas in which this interaction takes place, it is necessary for the nurse to assess various arenas. Any intervention in one arena will affect all other arenas.

3. Sorting should be under the categories listed below:

Life, Dignity, and Integrity Promoting:

Health benefits
Sick annual leave usable immediately
Possible advanced sick leave
Retirement plan
Disability insurance option

Positive Change Promoting:

Expectation to attend at least one in-service presentation per month
Sick employees wanting a challenge

Growth and Development Promoting:

Promotion consideration every two years
Payment of one-fourth to one-half tuition.
Able to apply for new position as available

Organizational Patterns:

University Medical Center consists of university hospital facilities

Acquiring and Using New Input:

Joint in-service medical facilities staff with university staff
Actively seeking new employees
Biannual promotion consideration

Assessment statement: The University Medical Center is a joint employment agency consisting of a university and medical facility. It seeks employees wanting a challenge and has employment policies that encourage continual growth and development of staff.

4. See Activity 2 for possible answers.
5. a. *life, dignity, and integrity:* police and fire departments; hospitals; emergency services, such as paramedics, poison control, and crisis centers; employment opportunities, and assistance for unemployed. Religious organizations; mortuaries; entertainment facilities; transportation and schools; communication systems, such as telephones, postal services, libraries, telegraphs, and newspapers; grocery stores; laundries; garbage disposal. Housing; stores for clothing and other items; banks and insurance companies; facilities for the handicapped, such as ramps, public restrooms, low telephones, etc.
   Remember to examine the accessibility of these services for the people who will need them.
   b. *positive change:* town meetings; local newspapers; voting mechanisms; arrangements for cross socioeconomic interactions for community members; local television and radio stations.
   c. *growth and development:* clubs for all ages; self-awareness groups; health education courses; continuing education courses; schools; medical services, such as physical and occupational therapy, optometrists; libraries; mental health services; banks.
   d. *organizational pattern:* villages, cities, townships, counties, wards, parishes, boroughs, or communes. Each has a different organizational pattern that permits the community to attain its purposes (goals).
   e. *acquiring and using new information:* newspaper; radio; television (local stations); new residents; schools; awareness groups; political system; public hearings.

© 1977 Wiley

PART I
STRESS AND STRAIN

INTRODUCTION

Research in the area of psychosocial needs and their effect on health, while tentative, suggests connections that are useful for professional nurses as they strive to render a service focused on moving the whole person toward optimum health. Psychosocial needs emerge from the client, his perceptions and feelings, significant others who interact with the client, and the stress normally encountered as one moves through life. When the client's psychosocial needs are met, recovery time from the disequilibrium of illness is reduced.

The nurse must be able to evaluate from available data the demands with which the client must cope, his coping capacity, and the external support available.

This module will introduce the learner to the assessment of the client's psychosocial needs. Clients are human beings who are subject to the normal stresses and potential inherent strain of living. Under conditions of illness and hospitalization, the client's usual coping pattern may not be sufficient to contain the stress and strain produced. Strain may be bearable when there is an active support system on which to lean.

When stress and strain are extensive, coping capacity low, and the support system inadequate, the client will need the nurse's active intervention to help him deal with the stress, which will free energy to regain health.

Assessment of the client's psychosocial needs is in keeping with the emphasis on the nurse's role in the maintenance of positive psychological health while the client has need of professional nursing care.

Basically, the nurse will need to assess the following three areas:

1. the stress and potential strain
2. the coping response
3. the support system

Nursing responsibility is to reduce overwhelming stress by foreseeing it and preparing the client in advance; to promote productive coping to stress by reinforcing and enchancing successfull patterns or teaching new ways to cope; and to facilitate active involvement of any available support system.

Upon successful completion of this module, the learner will have the knowledge that is basic to the psychosocial assessment of the client in relation to stress-strain, coping, and the importance of a support system. Prerequisites that would aid the learner in understanding the content are a course in general psychology and basic communication and interviewing skills.

TERMINAL OBJECTIVES

At the completion of Part 1 the learner will be able to do the following:

1. Analyze a client situation for stress and strain by:
    a. identifying those stresses with a high probability to produce strain

© 1977 Wiley

PSYCHOSOCIAL ASSESSMENT **95**

    b. translating behavioral data into the concept of strain
    c. estimating the degree or level of strain behavior
2. Analyze a client situation for coping behaviors by distinguishing between productive and nonproductive coping behavior.
3. Analyze a client situation for the presence of an involved support system by:
    a. identifying characteristics for an adequate support system
    b. evaluating behaviors of the support system for its involvement with the client
    c. evaluating client response to the support system

ACTIVITY 1
ASSESSMENT OF STRESS AND STRAIN

DEFINITION OF TERMS
Stress: noxious stimuli that interfere with satisfaction of needs and produce disequilibrium.

Strain: the negative effects of stress on the person.

Coping: the response of the person in stress that attempts to reduce the stress and/or strain.

Support System: the interpersonal and community network in the person's life that assists him to reduce stress and/or strain.

    Stress is an individual affair. What is perceived as stressful for one person may be a challenge to another; that is, stress does not automatically evoke strain and distress in a linear fashion. Productive coping and an active support system are mediating factors.

    That a person is in stress may not be evident until signs and symptoms of strain appear. Strain expresses itself in a person's thoughts, feelings, and behavior. Thinking clearly may be difficult, as there is a lack of an ability to concentrate. The person may exhibit a distressed affect, may look frightened or anxious, may report feelings of helplessness, disorganization, and despair. There is a functional physiological disturbance such as insomnia, anorexia, and tension. In addition, a person in strain lacks a reserve for coping with additional stress that may occur. He may overreact to minor stress with crying, angry outbursts, demandingness, or a sense of rising tension.

    The strength of the stress needs to be assessed for its potential to produce strain. Changes, losses, and life-threatening situations are usually strong stress stimuli that will produce some degree of strain. Also, stresses may accumulate to produce strain. Changes in a person's life may evoke adaptive efforts that are faulty in kind and duration. This produces a strain that lowers bodily resistance and increases the probability of disease.

Activity

The accompanying social readjustment rating scale was developed as a way of quantifying stressful life events. This exercise will help you assess your own stress level and will familiarize you with what are considered to be stressful life events that you will be noting in the lives of your clients.

    a. Check the events listed on the scale that have occurred in your life in the past 12 months.
    b. Add the given values to get a total score.
    c. Compare your score to the table of scores.

© 1977 Wiley

TABLE 1.
Social Readjustment Rating Scale[1]

Life Event	Mean Value	Life Event	Mean Value
Death of Spouse	100	Son or Daughter Leaving Home	29
Divorce	73	Trouble with In-Laws	29
Marital Separation	65	Outstanding Personal Achievement	28
Jail Term	63	Wife Begins or Stops Work	26
Death of Close Family Member	63	Begin or End School	25
Personal Injury or Illness	53	Change in Living Conditions	24
Marriage	50	Revision of Personal Habits	23
Fired at Work	47	Trouble with Boss	20
Marital Reconciliation	45	Change in Work Hours or Conditions	20
Retirement	45	Change in Residence	20
Change in Health of Family Member	44	Change in Schools	19
Pregnancy	40	Change in Recreation	19
Sex Difficulties	39	Change in Church Activities	18
Gain of New Family Member	39	Change in Social Activities	17
Business Adjustment	39	Mortgage or Loan Less Than $10,000	17
Change in Financial State	38	Change in Sleeping Habits	16
Death of Close Friend	37	Change in Number of Family Get-Togethers	15
Change to Different Line of Work	36	Change in Eating Habits	15
Change in Number of Arguments with Spouse	35	Vacation	13
Mortgage over $10,000	31	Christmas	12
Foreclosure of Mortgage or Loan	30	Minor Violations of the Law	11
Change in Responsibilities at Work	29		

[1] Holmes, T. H., and Rahe, R. H. J., 1967.

Score   *Chance of Becoming Sick*

0–150   37%
151–300   51%
301–up   80%

d. Your total score measures the accumulation of changes in your life that can be stressful. Remember, your score is not a guarantee of illness, since there are mediating factors such as successful coping and effective support systems.

Begin to notice signs and symptoms of stress and strain in yourself, friends, relatives, and clients.

1. Using the checklist and write-in form as a way to organize data, answer the following questions.
    a. Inquire and note the number and type of changes that have occurred in the person's life during the past 12 months.
    b. What is the specific stress now? Does it involve change, loss, or threat to life? Observe and ask the person about his affective state. Are unpleasant affects present such as grief, anxiety, and despair?
    c. Observe for a while and ask the client about disruption of functioning. Is there anorexia, insomnia, or decreased ability to concentrate?
    d. Note and inquire about coping reserve. Are there sudden tearful breakdowns, increased motor activity, a sense of rising tension?
2. Review the checklist write-in form.
3. Write a summary statement that includes the number and types of stress and the resulting strain if present.

© 1977 Wiley

PSYCHOSOCIAL ASSESSMENT 97

PROGRESS CHECK

Read the following situation and use the checklist for assessing stress and strain. Check your answers with the sample provided.

Situation: Mr. G. has been hospitalized for six weeks. He is in a body cast which will be removed in two more weeks. He is a house painter who fell from a second-story window to the concrete pavement, sustaining multiple fractures of both legs and pelvis. The medical team feels that he will not be able to support the weight-bearing activities of his present occupation.

Upon your approach Mr. G. looks frightened. After talking awhile, he expresses how confused and helpless he feels. He does not question the team or ask for information. During the interview he suddenly begins to cry while talking about a particular member of the medical team. He feels that this team member treats him roughly.

You notice in his chart that usually medication is given for sleep and he wakes frequently during the night. It has been noted that his appetite is poor. There has been a weight decrease of 10 pounds since admission. It has also been noted that his father died six months ago.

Checklist Write-In Form for Assessing Stress and Strain
1. Stress
   a. Number and type: _____

   b. Current stress:
      lifestyle change _____
      loss _____
      threat to life _____
2. Strain
   a. Affect:
      considerable apprehension _____
      fright or anxiety _____
      dejection, hopelessness _____
   b. Functional disturbance:
      insomnia _____
      anorexia _____
      reduced concentration _____
      constipation _____
      headache _____
      lassitude _____
   c. Coping reserve:
      sudden crying _____
      rising tension _____
      angry outburst _____
      low frustration tolerance _____
3. Assessment statement:

© 1977 Wiley

98 NURSING ASSESSMENT

ANSWERS
1. b. Current stress:
      hospitalization
      father died six weeks ago
      bodily injury
2. Strain
   a. Affect:
      frightened
      feelings of helplessness
   b. Functional disturbance:
      confusion
      insomnia
      anorexia
   c. Crying
      rising tension
      low tolerance
3. Assessment statement: Mr. G is experiencing an accumulation of stress: loss of close family member, bodily injury, and a lifestyle change. Strain is present in his affect (fright and anxiety), in functional disturbances (insomnia, loss of appetite with weight, and some confusion), and in his coping reserve, which is low (sudden crying).

ACTIVITY 2
ASSESSMENT OF COPING

Coping is a person's response as he or she attempts to reduce stress and strain. This response needs to be assessed to determine if it is productive or nonproductive.

Productive coping is dealing with reality in a problem-solving way so that stress is reduced and basically worked through. The person will attempt to perceive reality as clearly as he or she can. He or she will be asking questions, seeking new information, and checking out his or her perceptions. He or she will talk about his or her feelings openly as a way of reducing tension. He or she will actively participate in the experience, assuming control over daily life events as he or she is able. He or she will plan a course of action and put it to work.

Productive coping leads to strengthening of the person, so that each succeeding stress experience has less and less ability to cause strain. Self-esteem is maintained and enhanced. There is a sense of growth and mastery.

Nonproductive coping is retreating from reality in order to avoid or minimize psychic pain. Tension is reduced through the use of defense mechanisms that contain the strain but may not permit the person to deal with the stress directly. The person may deny or distort reality. He or she will attempt to reduce strain by low-level coping patterns that are self-comforting, such as:

1. reassurance of touch, rhythm, sound (humming, rocking, cuddling, and patting)
2. oral behavior (eating, smoking, and chewing gum)
3. use of alcohol and drugs
4. retreating (goofing off, sleeping, fantasizing, and daydreaming)

The person will not participate fully in the prescribed care and will want others to make decisions for him or her.

Nonproductive coping leads to a lack of growth and mastery over dealing with stress. It may leave the person with unrealistic fears and rigid control over emotional expression.

© 1977 Wiley

Activity

1. Reread the section on "Assessment of Coping"; as you read, make a list of productive and nonproductive coping behaviors.

   Productive   *Nonproductive*

   a.
   b.
   c.
   d.

2. Recall a stressful situation in your life:
   a. Using the checklist, assess your stress-strain.

   b. In writing, describe the behavior that helped or did not help you deal with the stress.

   c. Using the above list, categorize your coping as productive or nonproductive.

3. Generate a set of questions that you might ask in order to obtain information about how other people cope. When you have completed this task, in writing, check your questions with the answer sheet.

4. Using the above questions, practice focusing on the area of coping by talking with others; then categorize the data as productive or nonproductive.

© 1977 Wiley

PROGRESS CHECK

Using the following questions assess a client in the area of stress and coping:

a. In a stressful situation, what are you feeling?
b. What do you think about?
c. In what way is your body affected?
d. What are some ways you deal with stress?
e. What works best for you to reduce tension that accompanies stress?
f. Some people try to avoid stress. What are some ways you do this?
g. What helps you to face stress directly and deal with it?

ACTIVITY 3
ASSESSMENT OF THE SUPPORT SYSTEM

Psychosocial factors can affect health both positively and negatively through covert physiological mechanisms and overt behaviors. A support system reduces the stress reaction in the body and facilitates physiological recovery. It also supports the active involvement of the client in his treatment and movement toward health. Rapid recovery from disease and disability seem to depend on two major psychological factors: ego strength and lack of depression. A strong and active support system will back up ego strength and will prevent loss of morale and depression. Every client needs a support system. This system is made up of people and their interactions with each other. The client feels when he is accepted as he is and is warmly cared for. The family generally is most able to do this, owing to the congruency of culture and belief system, as well as blood ties. Often overlooked is the importance of friendships and work relationships as support systems. In some instances the client may be separated from his support system. The nurse may assume this role to meet the client's need.

In order to give support a support system must actively relate to the client. Physical presence of the support system with the client is ideal and where possible should be arranged, especially for children. When physical presence is impossible, the use of the telephone makes involvement possible. An active support system facilitates the client's reestablishment of equilibrium by assisting with productive coping, decreasing stress, and decreasing feelings of isolation, powerlessness, and depression.

This area must be assessed for its adequacy to support and its active involvement with the client. Assessment will determine what actions will be required of the nurse in relation to the client's needs. If the support system is found to be lacking, possible nursing interventions might be to engage the system or to enlarge or change it. Interventions are not within the scope of this module and will not be discussed here.

In summary, an active support system will:

1. facilitate reestablishment of equilibrium
2. reduce recovery time from serious illness
3. facilitate growth and development
4. reduce stress and strain
5. promote undisturbed physiological processes
6. reduce susceptibility to physiological stress
7. help the client maintain self-esteem

© 1977 Wiley

Support systems are assessed by observing the behavior of the supporting individual(s) and the client as they interact and noting the subsequent effect on the client. The nurse may also interview the supportive person(s) directly. The client can also be asked what he feels after a visit from the supportive person(s). Behaviors of the supportive person(s) that demonstrate their involvement and adequacy include:

1. The system communicates information clearly. The system approaches the team for information or gives appropriate information when needed.
2. The system facilitates the client's verbalization of feelings. The system asks the client to state his feelings. The system stays with the client when he expresses strong emotions, rather than moving away as defensive systems sometimes do.
3. The system supports independence by encouraging the client to make his own decisions.
4. There is a feeling of warmth and closeness. The system expresses concern and shows caring for the client.
5. After contact with the support system, the client's responses are changed. The client exhibits less strain behavior, a more relaxed affected state, has less disturbed physiological processes, has more coping reserve, and evidences productive coping behavior.

PROGRESS CHECK

1. Recall a stressful situation in which you felt supported by others around you.
2. In writing, answer the following:
    a. Name the people who made up your support system.

    b. What was their relationship to you—family, friends, work, etc.

    c. State several behaviors of that system that helped you to reduce and deal with stress.

    d. If you can, state several behaviors that did not help you.

3. Review Activity 3 and compare your written answers to the behaviors listed.

© 1977 Wiley

PART II
ARENAS OF STRESS

INTRODUCTION

Psychosocial nursing concepts acknowledge the individual as an open system within the context of environment. The individual's interaction with his environment affects him and vice versa. The environment can be conceived of as having space and time. Space is the location of the individual in the world and universe; time is the point in history where that person exists as well as the point in present time. With the rate of change in societies today, present time encompasses the past ten years. Thus, when considering the individual, the nurse must be aware that because they both exist in *this* era, certain things are important. For example, anyone born after World War II can conceive of landing on the moon with less awe than someone born earlier. Another example is that individuals born after World War II have difficulty envisioning a depression. Women in the 1970s differ from those of the 1930s in part because the women's movement happened in the seventies. To go one step further, the changes in abortion laws, in available employment, and in credit-granting policies have occured in the seventies partially because of the women's movement. Hence the breadth of the concept of environment.

When considering environment, one commonly thinks only of the geographical context and weather conditions. In an earlier age these conditions had high priority for one's daily life. People have learned to live with the various geographical and weather conditions and to reduce their dangers to a minimum.

Another part of the environmental context is culture. Culture is the combination of symbols, mores, norms, values, and belief systems held by an individual or group. The organization and interrelatedness of these elements provide the character and uniqueness of each culture. The manifestations of culture exist in space in the form of symbols and behaviors; hence, culture is a part of the environment an individual occupies. Based on cultural preferences, people exist in groupings called families, communes, kibbutzes, or clans. Several communities together may be called a city. Multiple cities combine to become states, and states unite to form countries. Within these countries individuals gather as subgroups to perform necessary tasks. The organization of each of the groupings reflects the environmental context.

One can find the unique characteristics resulting from the environmental (space, time, geographical, and cultural) context for each group. For example, in an environment that requires the inhabitants to defend the group daily and to hunt for food daily, and in which death comes by the age of thirty, the cultural values might center around youth, strength, agility, and fertility. In a more stable environment where the future is predictable, housing is mass-produced, food is obtainable from a grocery store, and death is delayed till age seventy, the cultural values might center around providing for retirement and enjoyment of leisure. In each group the sense of security would be affected by the degree to which weapons had been developed. Also part of the environment would be the inhabitants' spiritual belief systems. All of these parts are important, as together they form the foundation for an individual's actions.

The previous Activity—on coping—focused on the many incidents and situations in an individual's life that can be stressful. These incidents occur in space contexts, which may be called arenas. An arena is a circumscribed area where interactions take place between the individual and the environment. Whether or not an incident is considered stressful depends on the individual's background—that is, his location in time and space. A nurse needs to continually be aware of the multiple arenas experienced by an individual.

The nurse may need to intervene in any of the various arenas of a client's environment, such as the home, employment, religion; educational, recreational, or health-care settings; and the

© 1977 Wiley

greater community. Interventions within any one arena will affect all other arenas. In order to intervene adequately and effectively the nurse needs to be able to assess each of the client's arenas. In this part of the module three arenas will be discussed: a functional arena—the family; a structured arena—a health-care setting; and a conceptual arena—the community.

TERMINAL OBJECTIVES

At the completion of Part 2 the learner will be able to:

1. identify examples of culture and arena
2. identify the parts of a process
3. identify purposes of a process
4. explain the need for an arena assessment
5. sort, categorize, and write an assessment statement for at least one arena
6. assess an agency from one's own neighborhood
7. generate a list of five ways an arena could meet the criteria, utilizing the five criteria questions for arena assessment

ACTIVITY 1
A FRAMEWORK FOR ASSESSING AN ARENA

The individual as an open system interacting with the environment implies a process. This process of interacting begins when the egg and sperm unite and continues until death. It is ever-changing, and it occurs in varying arenas. Since each process and arena is such an integral part of the individual's life, it is important to be able to assess the processes in each arena.

Bevis[2] claims a process has three components: (1) inherent *purpose* or reason for being; (2) internal *organization* or method for achieving goals; and (3) *innovation* or provision to receive and to use new input. No matter how small or large the system, these three components are present. The digestive system in the human being is a good example. Its purpose is to provide nourishment to the human being. Its organization consists of all the parts and enzymes, which carry out a step-by-step process. The food must go through each phase to be broken down into the forms usable by the body. Poorly chewed food means loss of nourishment, as the food is not prepared for the next step in the process.

The three arenas to be assessed in this module are the family, an agency, and the community. Each of these has purpose, organization, and innovation. Though each has the same primary purpose, the varying goals account for the difference in organization and innovation.

The primary purpose of any system is self-perpetuation. Bower's[3] criteria for priority setting for the individual family or community are (1) threats to life, dignity, and integrity, (2) threats of destructive change, and (3) threats to normal growth and development. These priorities can be reworded in terms of promoting positive change and promoting normal growth and development

---

[2] Bevis, Em Olivia, *Curriculum Building in Nursing: A Process*, 1973.
[3] Bower, Fay Louise, *The Process of Planning Nursing Care: A Practice Model*, 1976.

104 NURSING ASSESSMENT

TABLE 2
A Model for Assessing an Arena

Purpose	Organization	Innovation
Promotes life, dignity, and integrity	Functional pattern (the family)	Input
Promotes positive change	Structured pattern (the health-care agency)	Discussion
Promotes normal growth and development	Conceptual pattern (community)	Decisions

of an individual, family, or community. For example, both a family and a community can have the same positive purpose of promoting life, dignity, and integrity. Each has a different goal or way for meeting that purpose, and each has differing organizational patterns for reaching the goal. The family will promote life by procreation; the community will promote life by providing employment.

Although each arena can be analyzed in terms of function, structure, or conceptualization, certain arenas emphasize specific terms. The family has traditional *functions* for the individual. A business or agency survives by organizational *structure*. A community can be geographical, ideological, or spiritual; hence it is a *conceptual* system. Assessment for each system will be discussed in the next Activity.

Table 2 presents a model for assessment of arenas using the Bevis components of a process and the rewording of Bower's priorities. It is useful for conceptualization of the arena processes. Each arena has a different organizational plan with different ways for innovation, yet they all have the same purposes. The following Progress Check will review the material presented thus far.

PROGRESS CHECK

1. When we speak of the individual interacting with the environment, the two concepts that make up environment are _____ and _____.

2. Match the words from the list on the left under the categories on the right.

   Culture   *Arena*   *Process Components*   *Process Purpose*

   a. promotes growth and development
   b. family
   c. norms
   d. innovation
   e. belief system
   f. health-care facility
   g. values
   h. organization
   i. mores
   j. community
   k. promotes positive change
   l. school
   m. purpose
   n. promotes life, dignity, and integrity
   o. symbols

3. An arena is a circumscribed area in which _____ takes place between an individual and the environment.

4. Whether or not something is considered stressful to an individual depends on _____.

© 1977 Wiley

ANSWERS
1. space, time

2.
Culture	Arena	Process Components	Process Purpose
norms	family	innovation	Promotes growth and development
belief system	health-care facility	organization	promotes positive change
values	community		
symbols	school	purpose	promotes life, dignity, and integrity

3. interactions
4. the person's background or location in space and time

ACTIVITY 2
ARENA ASSESSMENT
Assessing a Functional System: The Family

The first step in making an assessment is to select the arena. The first arena to be assessed is the family.

FAMILY ASSESSMENT
A person's primary group is the family. Since the criteria for assessment of an arena include the presence of purpose, organization, and innovation, the assessment of the family arena will include answers to the following questions:

1. How does the family promote life, dignity, and integrity?
2. How does the family promote positive change?
3. How does the family promote normal growth and development?
4. What is the organizational pattern of this family?
5. How does the family acquire and use new information?

Data can be collected by interview, observation, reviewing records, and referring to the literature. An interview of each family member will give information about how each thinks the family meets the criteria. An interview with the total family group not only will supply answers to questions asked by the interviewer, but will provide an opportunity for observation of interactions. The interviewer can observe the process for demonstration of purpose, organization, and innovation. Family records exist in the form of pictures, documents, and stories. School records, clinical records, and financial records all contain information about the family arena. A review of the literature can provide information of a more general nature. For example, the literature is often a source of information about a particular cultural group, kinship pattern, or communication model.

Janet, Jerry, and Roberta are classmates in a nursing program. They have been assigned to a men's psychiatric unit. During a class conference they describe their clients, the diagnoses, and the clients' behaviors. The teacher writes the following data on the blackboard.

© 1977 Wiley

106 NURSING ASSESSMENT

Janet	*Jerry*	*Roberta*
Mr. Frank Gibson	Mr. George Mason	Mr. Antonio Ramirez
Diagnosis: Manic-Depression	Diagnosis: Manic-Depression	Diagnosis: Manic-Depression
Age: 42	Age: 42	Age: 42
Married	Married	Married
Three teen-agers	Three teen-agers	Three teen-agers
Wife, age 41; employed as secretary	Wife, age 41; employed as secretary	Wife, age 41; employed as secretary
Own home	Own home	Own home
Husband employed as insurance salesman	Husband employed as insurance salesman	Husband employed as insurance salesman
First hospitalization	First hospitalization	First hospitalization
Medication: Lithium 300 mg. q.i.d.	Medication: Lithium 300 mg. q.i.d.	Medication: Lithium 300 mg. q.i.d.

The students look at each other in surprise. It looks as though their clients are exactly the same. But they know that they are very different. They begin to explore the differences.

Janet: "Well, each man has different cultural background."
Roberta: "Yes, and Mr. Ramirez mentioned that his wife just started working six months ago."
Jerry: "Mrs. Mason has been working since their marriage. She was unemployed during the years while the children were preschool age."
Janet: "Now that you mention it, Mr. Gibson did say something about his wife always being busy working. And he said that his mother-in-law lives with them."

As the conversation continues, the students begin to see that in order to really understand their clients they need to know more about their positions in space and time. To plan appropriate interventions, they need to know about the cultural variables and the family arena. They decide to speak to their clients and their wives about a family conference. The conferences will be directed toward obtaining answers to the five questions listed at the beginning of this Activity.

At the next conference Janet, Jerry and Roberta report on their family conferences.

Janet

Mr. Gibson identifies himself as black-American. The family members share his cultural identification. Mr. Gibson and his children used to have many interesting conversations about black history and their heritage. They have been able to trace their ancestry back to 1830.

Mr. and Mrs. Gibson discuss family problems, but Mr. Gibson makes the final decisions. The children share their concerns with their mother, who then relays this information to her husband. Mrs. Gibson sees her husband as not being firm with the chil-

Jerry

Mrs. Mason identifies himself as white Irish Catholic. The family share his cultural identification. Mr. Mason is upset by the changes in the Liturgy of the Catholic church. His children, however, for the first time are enjoying attending church. John, the oldest son, invited a priest to the house to discuss the changes in the church. The priest explained that some churches in the diocese still held traditional services and left a list with the family.

Mr. and Mrs. Mason share the head-of-household position. They make all decisions

Roberta

Mr. Ramirez identifies himself as Mexican-American. His children prefer to be called Chicano. There used to be arguments between the father and his children over the use of the word Chicano. However, a long family conference resulted in agreement that they each could use which word they wanted. Mrs. Ramirez was instrumental in the family's having the conference. She explained that she had been reading some articles on La Raza and found them interesting.

Usually Mr. Ramirez makes all decisions. He's seen

© 1977 Wiley

dren. She says, "He gives them anything they want." The children think he's unfair because he makes them do the dishes, ironing, and clean the house. Mr. Gibson thinks that boys and girls need to learn these chores. He had to!

Mrs. Gibson's mother often provides a sympathetic ear for the various family members. She, too, makes her feelings known to her daughter. She receives a social security check each month and contributes $40 a month to the family income. Since her husband died she has spent her time working with the church organizations and visiting her friends. Sometimes she has her friends over for lunch when the rest of the family are not home. She doesn't want to be in the way. Mrs. Gibson says she's glad her mother's there because now she doesn't worry as much about the children. Her mother's there when they get home from school. Since her husband's hospitalization Mrs. Gibson's mother has been fixing dinner, which allows Mrs. Gibson to work overtime several nights a week. The extra money has been helpful. Although she's busy, Mrs. Gibson belongs to a social club. She also reads and sews for relaxation.

together. Mr. Mason just began spending money without consulting her. She has been able to make ends meet with her salary and didn't say anything about the spending for months. Last month she had to apply for a loan. She was thankful she subscribed to a women's magazine where she read an article about married women being able to borrow money without their husband's signature. She didn't want to stop the children's allowances, although she decreased the amount. She had a talk with the children explaining the need to change their allowances. The oldest son could still use the gas credit card, as he drove his brother and sister to their extracurricular activities and then picked them up.

Mrs. Mason has someone come to clean the house once a week. She does the cooking and washing. The things that need ironing are sent to the laundry.

Mrs. Mason returned to school last quarter. She's taking a course in business management. She hopes to be able to advance in her job. Last summer she took a course in macramé and has made several wall hangings for her home. She enjoys interior decorating.

as the head of the household and the main breadwinner. He's a high achiever and doesn't want his wife to work. He sees her responsibility as the house. The children help with the chores.

Both Mr. and Mrs. Ramirez's families live nearby. Mrs. Ramirez and the children have been eating more frequently at their relatives' homes. (This has helped to offset some of the family expenses.)

Mr. Ramirez's father had spoken to him several times about his spending habits. He tried to get his son to talk to a priest or to visit the local curandero. Mr. Ramirez ignored his father's request. Finally, Mrs. Ramirez saw an advertisement on television about the family crisis center. She called the number and made an appointment. The staff at the crisis center helped the family to get Mr. Ramirez to the hospital.

Mrs. Ramirez is friends with a few of her neighbors. She often gets together with them for a pot-luck dinner. There are some young couples on the street. The experienced women have been helping them learn to be "good" wives and learn childrearing practices.

Six months ago Mrs. Ramirez began working after completion of a special program at a local community college. The program is designed to help women who have been unemployed for many years to learn skills to reenter the job market.

108 NURSING ASSESSMENT

The next step in the assessment process is to sort and categorize the data using the criteria for family assessment. Below are Janet's data sorted and categorized.

Life, Dignity and Integrity Promoting

Discussion around black history and heritage
Grandmother has friends and works in church
Grandmother helps with child supervision and household chores
Grandmother contributes financially to family
Mrs. Gibson able to work overtime

Positive Change Promoting

Mother and grandmother approachable for discussion and sharing of problems
Flexibility for getting household chores done

Growth and Development Promoting

Ethnic identification agreement.
Children are expected to learn how to do household chores
Grandmother involved in community after husband's death
Family members can share problems with someone

Organizational Patterns

Mr. Gibson makes final decision.
Mr. and Mrs. Gibson discuss problems.
Mrs. Gibson receives communication on problems, then relays information to her husband
Children and grandmother follow decisions of Mr. Gibson

Acquiring and Using New Information

Information passes through mother to father
Father makes decisions after discussion with his wife

The final step is to write an assessment statement. The assessment statement for the Gibson family:

The Gibson family consists of three children, parents, and maternal grandmother. The family has a strong ethnic identification with black American culture. Mr. Gibson is currently hospitalized; however, his wife's employment is sustaining the family. Mr. Gibson is acknowledged as the head of the household and makes all decisions with his wife's input. Mrs. Gibson and grandmother support other family members' coping ability. New information is filtered through Mrs. Gibson to Mr. Gibson. The grandmother is a widow, has interest in and outside the home.

PROGRESS CHECK

1. Sort and categorize Jerry's data.

© 1977 Wiley

2. Write an assessment statement.

ANSWERS
1. Below are the categories used and data sorted for the Mason family.

Life, Dignity, and Integrity Promoting

Children are enjoying and attending church
Mr. and Mrs. Mason share head-of-household responsibility
Mr. and Mrs. Mason employed.
Mrs. Mason has outside assistance with household chores
Mr. Mason expressing his religious sermon preferences and learning alternatives

Positive Change Promoting

Discussion with priest.
Mother discussed need to reduce allowance amount
Mrs. Mason applies information learned in school (macramé)

Growth and Development Promoting

Children receive allowance.
Children learn to manage a financial decrease
Mrs. Mason attending school to increase skills.
Shared religious identification.
Children participate in extracurricular activities

Organizational Pattern

Mr. and Mrs. Mason make all decisions together
Oldest brother has responsibility toward younger siblings

Acquiring and Using Information

Discussion of area of discontent.
Mrs. Mason read magazine article, later recalled information and acted on it

2. Assessment statement: The Mason family consists of three children and two parents. During Mr. Mason's hospitalization, Mrs. Mason's income is supporting the family. The need to borrow money has been shared with the family members. Mr. and Mrs. Mason make decisions together. Family discussions are held for problems. Children have no household responsibility but oldest has responsibility for siblings getting to and from extracurricular activities. The family practices Catholicism.

Assessing a Structured System: An Agency

A structured system can be a small business, a large corporation, or a public agency. It can be a health-care facility or a school. An assessment of a structured system follows the same steps as the family assessment. Once you decide on which system, apply the criteria. In this instance data for the following questions would be collected:

1. How does this system promote life, dignity, and integrity?
2. How does this system promote positive change?
3. How does this system promote normal growth and development?
4. What is the organizational pattern of this system?
5. How does the system acquire and use new information?

PROGRESS CHECK

Select a health-care facility in your neighborhood (a neighborhood health clinic, prenatal clinic, well baby clinic, women's clinic, free clinic, or hospital). Visit the agency and begin gathering data on the above questions. Remember, you need to look at the agency from the perspective of the consumer and from that of the employees. (Thus this serves as an assessment tool for a prospective employer.)

You can begin to gather data by reading any handouts or literature printed by the agency. A statement of the agency's philosophy is usually available. This will provide beginning answers to your questions. A review of recent newspapers may contain articles about the agency. What type of advertising does the agency use? Most agencies have a public relations officer or a director, who may be willing to speak with the public. A telephone call requesting an appointment, stating that you are a student, is often enough to gain entry. As you obtain your data, sort and categorize them under the categories below.

Life, Dignity and Integrity Promoting   *Positive Change Promoting*   *Growth and Development Promoting*

Organizational Patterns   *Acquiring and Using New Information*

ANSWERS

Life, Dignity and Integrity

Lifesaving devices, diagnostic procedures, medications, health professionals, concern for privacy, explaining treatments to clients, not allowing a person to do something that he or she would later be ashamed of, considering the client's background, needs, and preferences.

Health teaching or community outreach staff, an in-patient facility, a chapel or provision for religious services for the clients. Etc.

Positive Change Promoting

Health teaching, family groups, self-help groups, consumer information, community forums, open houses.

Growth and Development Promoting

Diagnostic procedures, physical and occupational therapy, emergency rooms, immunizations, prenatal courses self-awareness groups.

Organizational Pattern

A pyramid where all decisions are made at the top and filtered down. It might have several de-

Acquiring and Using New Information

In-service programs, community forums, consumer input, suggestion boxes.

© 1977 Wiley

partments. There may be several management positions. It could have a team format, where each member has an equal input in decision making. There may be a citizen's advisory group or a board of directors.

The development of new equipment, new staff. The decisions around the use of information may depend upon the board of directors, policies, the agency director, or group consensus.

An assessment statement would mention each criterion and what was found for that agency. For example, the Springtown Free Clinic provides emergency services for all in need, regardless of age or financial status. It provides a series of on-going prenatal and exercise courses. It has referral services to other community agencies. It holds a monthly forum on consumer issues. The clinic is organized in six teams, each with a client caseload. A board of directors makes policy. New information is discussed by the board of directors, and recommendations are made to the teams. The six teams vote. Majority vote decides.

Assessing a Conceptual System: The Community

The third arena of assessment is that of the community. We will need to ask the same criteria questions we used before.

1. How does the community promote life, dignity, and integrity?
2. How does the community promote change?
3. How does the community promote normal growth and development?
4. What is the organizational pattern of the community?
5. How does the community acquire and use new information?

PROGRESS CHECK

To begin, select a radius of ten city blocks or five miles. A walk or drive through this area should begin the assessment process. Take along a road map, or draw a map, and mark the location of various services and the residences. In a small community the telephone book will provide easy access to community agencies. Interviewing residents will give information about their perception of the community's ability to meet the criteria. Local newspapers will have information about any community development plans and other community issues. Many cities now have a specific magazine, e.g., *San Francisco, Phoenix, Augusta.* Look to see if the city to be assessed has such a magazine.

The community organizational pattern and political system will also need to be assessed. Whether or not a community is a village or city makes a difference for the services it has and its relationship to the state political system; likewise for other categories, such as townships or parishes. A community can have different services based on the county in which it exists. Does the community have a mayor? Is there a citizens advisory board or board of supervisors? What is their relationship to the community?

Also there may be neighborhood organizations. Neighborhoods where there is a lot of crime may form local surveillance teams. Sometimes there are block organizations for such projects as street lighting, trees, street clean-up and repair. A community may have a

© 1977 Wiley

helping-friend system. This service is often extended through religious organizations for the elderly and/or infirm.

Where are the stores for food and clothing? Where are housing facilities in relationship to stores and health-care facilities? What types of transportation are available? Do most members of the community have automobiles? Is there a public transportation system? Is there a taxicab or jitney service? Do these services ease at a certain hour? Do these health-care agencies have ambulances, or is a private ambulance company needed? Does the health-care agency provide transportation for clients?

What provisions are there for communication? What percentage of community members have radio, television, or receive a daily paper? Is there a local newspaper, radio, or television station? Are public telephones available in the streets rather than in business establishments? Are they in operating order?

What type of housing is available? Is the housing around areas mixed culturally and across age lines? If not, is there any group with no housing or very limited housing?

Is entertainment available? What types? Does the community have playgrounds, recreation centers, zoos, museums, movies, playhouses, etc.? What is the ratio of entertainment facilities to age groups? Is any age group omitted? Are there ways for expression of cultural, ethnic, or religious preferences?

What opportunities exist in the community for employment or assistance for the unemployed? Is a community college nearby? Do the schools offer adult education courses? Does the television station offer college courses? What types of businesses exist in the community?

Is there a police force? What emergency services does it offer? How large is it? Is the fire department salaried or voluntary? Does the city have a paramedic emergency service?

A lot of questions need to be asked to get a community assessment. Once the data are acquired, the nurse will find them invaluable in planning health care. A community assessment also offers benefits to every individual. A person's understanding of the community can enhance one's interaction within it.

You have finished this module on Psychosocial Assessment. The Posttest with answers will help you evaluate what you have learned. If you have any difficulty answering the questions, review the module or consult your instructor. If you cannot answer all the questions, review the module until you can.

POSTTEST

PART 1
Read the situation and answer the questions that follow.

Situation: Mr. F. is a 22-year-old married man, father of a three-year-old boy. He was hospitalized for a crushing injury to his right hand, sustained on his job as a machine operator. The treatment consisted of an emergency surgical amputation of four fingers and three reconstructive surgeries during the past month.

Mr. F. consented to talk with the nurse about his illness and hospitalization, saying, "It's good to get it off your chest." He appeared friendly although in mild pain. He knew a great deal about his treatment and was cooperative in the daily hospital routine. He looked worried at times but overall did not appear depressed. He smoked more than usual. He has some difficulty sleeping. His appetite is normal and weight is maintained.

He misses his wife and son and keeps a picture of his family on the bedside table. The family home is a hundred miles from the large urban hospital. His wife drives to the hospital each

114 NURSING ASSESSMENT

weekend to stay with him. After each visit Mr. F. has a brighter affect and sleeps better during the night.

He worries about how others will respond to his injured hand. He examines it himself, and he showed it to his wife, who reacted with acceptance. He is verbalizing his grief and anger in reaction to his changed body image.

In the hospital he directs his care by suggesting ways his cast can be made more comfortable. He visits often with other patients on the ward.

Although he will not be able to return to his old job, he is making plans to study accounting at a local college. He had little emotional investment in his old job. He feels his new career will be more interesting and personally satisfying.

1. What is the specific stress? (Order with highest stress first.)

2. Is there evidence of strain? Give behavioral data to substantiate your answer.

3. Is coping productive or nonproductive? Give behavioral data to substantiate your answer.

4. What is the support system and is it active and effective? Give behavioral data to support your answer.

© 1977 Wiley

PART 2

1. The three parts of a process are _____, _____, and _____.

2. The purposes of a process are:
   a. _____
   b. _____
   c. _____

3. Examples of arenas are _____, _____, and _____.

4. Culture is a complicated concept. It consists of: _____, _____, _____, and _____.

5. Which of the following is an acceptable reason for doing an arena assessment?
   a. Arena is another word for family. Everyone exists in a family setting. The nurse needs to know about the family setting.
   b. An arena is an individual's community. Rather than making interventions on an individual level, the nurse must begin making only community interventions, that is, to be able to assess the arena.
   c. Arenas are areas where the individual and his environment interact. The nurse needs to know about these interactions, as change in one affects all others.

6. Review Activity 2. Using the data on the Ramirez family:
   a. Sort, and categorize:

   b. Write an assessment statement:

© 1977 Wiley

116 NURSING ASSESSMENT

7. Explore your neighborhood. Consider a ten-block or five-mile radius. Make an assessment of the community.

8. Below are the five criteria questions for assessment of a health-care facility from the standpoint of *an employee*. List at least five ways a health-care facility could meet the criteria.
   a. How does the health-care facility promote life, dignity, and integrity?

   b. How does the health-care facility promote positive change?

   c. How does the health-care facility promote growth and development?

   d. What is the organizational plan of the health-care facility?

   e. How does the health-care facility acquire and use new input?

© 1977 Wiley

Answers

PART 1

1. a. *loss* of function of right hand
   b. *change* of body image
   c. *change* of future employment
2. Give behavioral data.
   a. yes, mild strain
   b. data: worried or distressed affect
      smoking more to reduce felt tension
      functional disturbance: difficulty sleeping
3. Give behavioral data to substantiate your answer.
   a. coping is productive.
   Data: Verbalizes feelings as a way of reducing tension; "It's good to get it off your chest;" verbalizes grief and anger; has coping reserve: friendly although in mild pain; involved in experience: knew a great deal about his treatment; reality testing: Examines own hand, showed it to wife; maintains control over daily care: suggests ways his cast could be made more comfortable; lack of depression: friendly affect, outgoing, visits other patients; makes plan for future: plans to go to school and change employment.
4. Give behavioral data to support your answer.
   a. Support system consists of wife and son.
   b. Active: Wife makes arrangements to drive a hundred miles to spend weekends with patient.
   c. Effectiveness: After each visit the patient's affect is brighter; functional disturbance is reduced; and the patient sleeps better.

PART 2

1. purpose, organization, innovation
2. a. promote life, dignity, and integrity
   b. promote positive change
   c. promote growth and development
3. family, health-care facility, community
4. mores, values, norms, belief systems
5. c.
6. a.

Life, Dignity and Integrity Promoting	*Positive Change Promoting*	*Growth and Development Promoting*
Mr. and Mrs. Ramirez employed	Use of discussion to explore different opinions about Chicano versus Mexican-American	Identification with ethnic group and label consistent with ideology of age groups
Mrs. Ramirez's employment and extended family members help family during Mr. Ramirez's hospitalization	Family able to seek help from community agency	Mrs. Ramirez gets together with her friends for pot-luck dinners. The women share their knowledge and experience with other women.

Organization Pattern		*Acquiring and Using New Information*
Mr. Ramirez is head of household, makes all decisions		Mrs. Ramirez's reading articles on La Raza encouraged family discussion

© 1977 Wiley

Mrs. Ramirez's domain is household. Children help mother with chores
Extended family members, living nearby, support family when needed

An advertisement by local mental health association on television led Mrs. Ramirez to contact the family crisis center

b. Assessment Statement: Mr. Ramirez is presently hospitalized. During this time the family is being sustained by his wife's employment and extended family assistance. Although Mr. Ramirez as head of household makes all decisions, he is willing to discuss topics with family members. The family members have similar ethnic identification, differing only along ideological lines. From television and reading the family members obtain information that is applied for their benefit.

7. Activity 2 in Part 2 of this module for possible answers. Also see answer 5 in the Pretest.

8. *Life, Dignity, and Integrity Promoting*

   1. Health-care and insurance plans (include disability and life insurance)
   2. Some autonomy for each person's job
   3. Employee health facilities
   4. On-the-job safety campaigns
   5. Concern for privacy

   Positive Change Promoting

   1. Staff get-togethers.
   2. Encourage supervisor/supervisee interaction other than around problems
   3. Suggestion box
   4. Communication workshops
   5. Grievance procedures

   Growth and Development Promoting

   1. Partial or full payment of tuition at local college
   2. Health-care plans with dental, optometry, and preventive health services
   3. Time off job for community involvement.
   5. In-service programs
   6. Office club/recreation teams
   7. On-site recreation exercise facilities

   Organization Pattern

   1. Small units where staff can get to know each other
   2. Team plan where each individual can have input
   3. Committees for problem solving
   4. Board of directors with community representatives from health and insurance companies
   6. Flexible work hours
   7. Constructive criticism and recognition for well-done job
   8. Attention to morale needs for job satisfaction
   9. Union representation

   Acquiring and Using New Information

   1. Company newspaper
   2. In-service programs
   3. Staff meetings
   4. Community outreach, e.g., open house, forums
   5. Contests

References

Holmes, T. H., and Rahe, R. H. J., *Psychosomatic Research* 2 (1967): 214.

Bevis, Em Olivia, *Curriculum Building in Nursing: A Process.* St. Louis: C. V. Mosby, 1973, pp. 8–9.

Bower, Fay Louise, *The Process of Planning Nursing Care: A Practice Model.* St. Louis: C. V. Mosby, 1976, p. 14.

LOIS M. HOSKINS, R.N., M.S.

WILEY NURSING CONCEPT MODULE

THE NURSING DIAGNOSIS

CONTENTS

    PRETEST 121   Answers 123

    INTRODUCTION 123

    TERMINAL OBJECTIVES 124

        ACTIVITY 1. The Problem-Solving Process 124
        ACTIVITY 2. Needs 125
        ACTIVITY 3. Patient Problems 127
        ACTIVITY 4. Nursing Intervention 128
        ACTIVITY 5. The Nursing Diagnosis 129

    POSTTEST 136   Answers 139

    REFERENCES 140

    SUGGESTED READINGS 140

© 1977 Wiley

PRETEST

If you are able to complete this pretest with 100% mastery, you do not need to study this module on nursing diagnosis.

Multiple Choice: Circle the letter of the one best answer.

1. Needs can *best* be described as:
    a. necessities for living
    b. something required for survival
    c. arranged in a hierarchical order
    d. something required for physical well-being

2. The nursing diagnosis is:
    a. the derivation of the patient's need from a situation
    b. identification of a health problem
    c. a summary statement of the patient's problem and its cause
    d. none of the above

3. Elimination, modification, or prevention of patient problems describes the:
    a. goal of nursing intervention
    b. outcomes in terms of patient behavior
    c. nursing actions
    d. last step in nursing diagnosis

4. In the context of the nursing diagnosis the patient problem is:
    a. a medical problem
    b. any problem the person might have
    c. a health-related problem
    d. a social problem

5. Which of the following occurs first?
    a. need
    b. patient problem
    c. nursing diagnosis
    d. nursing intervention

6. Which of the following statements describe actual patient problems?
    1. existing and operating in the situation
    2. anticipated from the condition
    3. may be described as a sign, symptom, or set of existing conditions
    4. likely to develop
        a. 2, 4
        b. 1, 3
        c. 2, 3
        d. 1 only

7. The main function of the nursing diagnosis is to:
    a. give direction to the plan of nursing care
    b. indicate the patient problem and its cause
    c. imply the unmet needs of the patient
    d. relate the goals and expected outcome of nursing intervention

8. The first step in making the nursing diagnosis is:
    a. identifying the patient need
    b. collecting the data base
    c. summarizing the data
    d. indicating the problem

© 1977 Wiley

122 NURSING ASSESSMENT

9. Loss of a body part for any reason will threaten one's body image. In this statement which of the following relationships are true?
   1. Threatened body image is the problem.
   2. Body image is the need.
   3. Loss of a body part is the problem.
   4. Loss of a body part is the cause of the problem.
      a. 2, 3, 4
      b. 2, 3
      c. 1, 2
      d. 1, 2, 4

10. In the following list put N in front of the Need and P in front of the Patient Problem:
    ____a. sleep
    ____b. abdominal distention
    ____c. loss of feeling of self-worth
    ____d. self-respect
    ____e. pain
    ____f. inability to communicate

11. Check the best examples of nursing diagnoses in the following:
    ____a. acute pancreatitis
    ____b. headache due to anxiety
    ____c. nausea and vomiting
    ____d. lack of self-confidence due to parental rejection
    ____e. chronic renal failure
    ____f. elevated white cell count related to appendicitis
    ____g. shortness of breath due to pain of surgical incision
    ____h. depression

12. Analyze the following situations:
    a. Summarize the data into a well-stated nursing diagnosis.
    b. State the indicated nursing intervention and the goals in terms of patient outcome.

    Situation 1: Janice, a 20-year-old college student, is admitted to the hospital for fever of unknown origin. She cries frequently and sleeps poorly. She tells you that next week is final test week and she has a paper due. You talk to her and she says, "I'm so worried—I don't know what is going to happen to me."

    Situation 2: A 70-year-old man has a history of congestive heart failure. He has been on diuretics for fluid retention. You observe that he has 3+ pitting edema about both ankles. He states that his feet feel puffy and heavy.

© 1977 Wiley

Answers

1. a 2. c 3. a 4. c 5. a 6. c 7. a 8. b 9. d
10. a. N b. P c. P d. N e. P f. P
11. b, d, f, g
12. Analysis of situations:

    Situation 1:
    a. *Nursing diagnosis.* Anxiety due to fear of unknown with respect to her illness and how it will influence her college situation.
    b. *Nursing intervention and patient outcomes.* The problem is anxiety, which is interfering with Janice's needs for safety and security. Intervention would be directed to the cause, fear of unknown with respect to her illness and how it will influence her college situation. The nurse would give Janice support and guidance by listening to her, being with her, and also by discussing her priorities with her. Her immediate priority is to determine the cause of the illness, initiate cure, and then direct her energies toward her college situation. The expected patient outcome is decreased anxiety.

    Situation 2:
    a. *Nursing diagnosis.* Edema of ankles due to decreased circulation due to congestive heart failure.
    b. *Nursing intervention and patient outcomes.* The problem is edema, which is interfering with this man's physiological needs and is indicative of more severe physiological problems (congestive heart failure). Intervention would be directed to the cause, decreased circulation due to congestive heart failure. The nurse would provide measures to improve circulation: TED stockings, elevation of extremities, etc. She would also treat congestive heart failure by moderation of diet and activity, observation and recording of signs and symptoms, support of medical regimen, etc. The expected patient outcome is reduction or elimination of the edema with improved circulation and stabilization of the heart condition.

INTRODUCTION

This module is designed to help you to understand how to make nursing diagnoses. It is divided into five Activities: (1) The Problem-Solving Process, (2) Needs, (3) Patient Problems, (4) Nursing Intervention, and (5) The Nursing Diagnosis. Each Activity has a text followed by exercises that enable you to develop mastery of the content. These Activities build on each other in sequential fashion and so should be studied in the order given. The self-tests for mastery proceed from basic levels of understanding of information to higher levels incorporating the ability to utilize the information in complex situations.

You have taken a pretest: there is also a posttest. If you score 100% on the pretest, you do not need to do the module. It would be desirable but not necessary for you to have knowledge of the problem-solving process prior to working on the module.

You may study alone, but it is suggested that you have one or more partners. In this way you may discuss the content with each other, ask each other questions, and apply the concepts to your own experiences. You will need no materials other than this module. It will probably be most effective if you plan to do the module in one sitting.

© 1977 Wiley

124 NURSING ASSESSMENT

TERMINAL OBJECTIVES

Upon completion of the module you will be able to do the following:

A. Given a set of test items or conditions, you will be able to:
 1. identify statements that describe need, patient problem, nursing intervention, and nursing diagnosis.
 2. distinguish between needs and problems.
 3. arrange, in order, the procedural steps in making a nursing diagnosis.
 4. identify statements that describe actual and potential patient problems.
 5. select statements describing the functions of nursing diagnoses.
 6. identify statements that describe the criteria for a well-stated nursing diagnosis.
 7. discuss needs and problems in your own life.

B. Given patient situations or statements describing patient conditions (needs, problems, nursing interventions, and nursing diagnoses), you will be able to:
 1. identify and explain the relationship between need, patient problem, and nursing intervention.
 2. prescribe the nursing intervention as derived from the nursing diagnosis.
 3. compare and evaluate statements of nursing diagnoses.
 4. analyze the given situation and formulate the nursing diagnosis.

ACTIVITY 1

THE PROBLEM-SOLVING PROCESS

In order to make a nursing diagnosis you must be able to problem-solve; that is, you must be able to define, describe, and utilize the steps of the problem-solving process. Write here or on a separate sheet of paper the steps of the problem-solving process and describe them. Compare them to those listed below.

© 1977 Wiley

THE NURSING DIAGNOSIS

STEPS OF THE PROBLEM-SOLVING PROCESS

1. Collection of data—gathering of information. In the context of the client[1] situation this would be information about the health status of the individual, family, or community involved.
2. Definition of the problem—decision arising from analysis of the data stating the difficulty or expressed concern.
3. Planning—identifying solutions to treat the problem.
4. Testing the plan—implementing the actions outlined in the plan.
5. Evaluation—judging the effectiveness of the actions taken to solve the problem.

Are you experiencing any problems right now? Are you or your partner in this learning experience having any difficulties or meeting any obstacles in fulfilling some requirement of yours? Discuss these and list characteristics of the difficulty here. Would they include any of the items below?

"I don't want to do this."
"I have a date."
"This is boring and time consuming."
"I'm hungry."
"I have a million things to do."

Do you have a problem? What is it? Is it the requirement to study this material? Continue the module and reassess your situation later.

ACTIVITY 2

NEEDS

Webster defines need as "necessity, lack of something required or desired."[2] Maslow[3] has postulated a hierarchy of basic human needs. These include:

1. Physiological needs—Survival needs, including nutrition, respiration, and elimination; sexual needs; desire for rest, activity, and comfort.
2. Safety needs—Freedom from fear or threat to either physical or psychosocial well-being.
3. Love needs—Need for affection or sense of belonging, a "place within his group."
4. Esteem needs—Need for good evaluation of self. Self-respect, self-confidence. Self-worth based on recognition by others.
5. Self-actualization needs—Need to be the most that one can be, life fulfillment.

---

[1] Client—relates to an individual, family, or community seeking health care. It incorporates the term "patient."
Patient—relates to an individual who is confined to a hospital or an institutional setting because of a health problem.
[2] *Webster's New World Dictionary of the American Language*, 1973.
[3] Maslow, A. H., *Motivation and Personality*, 1954.

© 1977 Wiley

He ranks these in order, stating that when one set of needs are met, a person then moves on to fulfilling the next higher set of needs. Thus when our physiological needs are met we can then consider our safety needs, when our safety needs are met we can consider our love needs, etc., up the order. An individual can be involved in meeting several different needs at one time. In some situations, such as those that are threatening, lower-level needs may assume more importance, at least temporarily.

Many factors influence a person's needs. Among these are:

1. age
2. sex
3. family and peer-group relationships
4. developmental status
5. past experience
6. health state (including physical, mental, and emotional state)
7. coping patterns
8. culture
9. occupation
10. finances
11. religion
12. demographic factors

These factors are likely to influence the level of need most significant in a particular situation. The amount of need may vary. An infant's needs or the means to fulfill them will vary from those of an adult. A successful writer who has just sustained a heart attack will find his self-actualization needs secondary to survival needs as his health state is threatened.

Identify your position in Maslow's hierarchy of needs. Which needs are most predominant in your life?

Are your survival needs fairly well satisfied? Probably they are—you are not in a daily struggle to obtain food, water, and oxygen.

How about your safety needs? Are you in a relatively new situation, encountering changes or something that threatens your usual physical and mental stability? As a college student you are in such a situation, so these needs might be greater than the physiological needs.

How about love and belonging needs? They are probably very great right now, too. You probably have an urge to belong, to have friends, and to be one of the group.

Consider the other needs in like manner.

Where do you place the need to study?

ACTIVITY 3
PATIENT PROBLEMS

The individual exists in a state of physiological and psychosocial equilibrium based upon the fulfillment and regulation of his or her basic needs. This state of equilibrium is the state of wellness or optimum health. Anything that threatens or disturbs this equilibrium may cause a change in the individual's health state that threatens his being. This constitutes a health problem. Therefore, the *patient problem*[4] may be defined as *anything that interferes or threatens to interfere with the patient's satisfaction and regulation of his needs.*

These problems may be further defined according to Bower[5] as occurring "when a client, family, or community:

1. cannot meet a need
2. needs help to meet a need
3. is not aware of an unmet need
4. has a conflict of apparently equally important needs
5. must choose from several alternative ways of meeting needs."

A list of patient problems based on this definition might appear as follows:

		Need	*Problem*
1.	Cannot meet a need	Adequate nutrition or food	Lack of money to buy food
2.	Needs help to meet a need	Adequate respiration	Irregular breathing pattern
3.	Is not aware of an unmet need	Maintenance of blood sugar balance	Diabetes—lack of knowledge of disease and its complications
4.	Has a conflict of apparently equally important needs	Need for rest, for exercise, socializing, and self-improvement	Lack of plan or schedule to include all of these
5.	Must choose from several alternative ways of meeting needs	Needs as item 4	Doesn't like known alternatives Lack of knowledge of all possible alternatives Lack of knowledge of how to compare alternatives

PROGRESS CHECK

Next to each statement write N for need, P for patient problem, and 0 for neither.

____ 1. taking a drink of water
____ 2. talking to your friends
____ 3. being sick every weekend
____ 4. going to a movie
____ 5. being hugged by someone you love

---

[4] *Patient problem* could also be stated *client problem*. Patient problem is the term most often encountered in the references. You are advised to use the terminology of your school.

[5] Bower, Fay Louise, *The Process of Planning Nursing Care: A Practice Model*, 1976.

© 1977 Wiley

____6. having $50 as your sole monthly income
____7. crying yourself to sleep every night
____8. being praised by a respected teacher

ANSWERS
1. N   2. N   3. P   4. 0   5. N   6. 0[6]   7. P   8. N

Now reassess your own situation. Look back at your statements at the end of Activity 1 and look at your needs as you stated them at the end of Activity 2. Did you call the requirement to study this material a need or a problem? Hopefully you said that by studying this material you would be able to make nursing diagnoses, which is a necessary goal for you if you are to become a professional nurse. Becoming a professional nurse helps meet your need of self-actualization. Probably if you have a problem (and you may not) it can be classified as a conflict of apparently equally important needs because of inadequate organization of time. Is this a health problem—is it going to threaten or interfere with your physiological and psychosocial equilibrium? Is this a problem you can solve by yourself? Do you need help? Consider these questions or discuss them with your partner.

ACTIVITY 4
NURSING INTERVENTION

Nurses intervene in patient problems. To intervene is "to come or be between, to modify, settle or hinder some action, etc."[7] Therefore, *the goal of nursing intervention is the elimination, modification, or prevention of patient problems* so that the patient's needs can be met. Relating this to Bower's problem statement in Activity 3, if the patient cannot meet a need, the nurse can do it for him; if he needs help to meet a need, the nurse can support him; if he is not aware of an unmet need, the nurse can teach him; if he needs help in making a decision, the nurse can guide him; and finally the nurse can alter the situation or environment to make the need satisfaction easier for him. Finding the solution to the patient's problem becomes a problem for the nurse.

PROGRESS CHECK

Return to the list of patient problems in Activity 3. Add another column entitled Nursing Intervention. What nursing intervention is indicated for each of the patient problems? Are your answers similar to those below?

ANSWERS

	Need	Patient Problem	Nursing Intervention
1. Cannot meet a need	Adequate nutrition or food	Lack of money to buy food	Refer to social worker
2. Needs help to meet a need	Adequate respiration	Irregular breathing pattern	Assist with breathing exercises
3. Is not aware of an unmet need	Maintenance of blood sugar balance	Diabetes—lack of knowledge of disease	Teach about diabetes and related health care

[6] This is a problem, and it may cause a health problem if no other source of food, clothing, and shelter exists.
[7] *Webster's New World Dictionary of the American Language,* 1973.

© 1977 Wiley

4. Has a conflict of apparently equally important needs	Need for rest, for exercise, socializing, and self-improvement	Lack of plan or schedule to include all of these	Assist with making activity schedule
5. Must choose from several alternative ways of meeting needs	Needs as item 4	Doesn't like known alternatives Lack of knowledge of all possible alternatives Lack of knowledge of how to compare alternatives	Provide further information to help explore possibilities of need fulfillment Suggest alterations in situation

ACTIVITY 5
THE NURSING DIAGNOSIS

Patient problem and nursing intervention have been defined. Now, what is nursing diagnosis? Webster[8] defines diagnosis as "the act of deciding the nature of a disease, situation, problem, etc. by examination and analysis; the resulting decision." *Nursing diagnosis is the definition of those patient problems amenable to nursing intervention.* Or, as stated by Gebbie and Lavin,[9] the nursing diagnosis is "the identification of those patient problems or concerns most frequently identified by nurses ... which are amenable to some intervention which is available in the present or potential scope of nursing practice."

How does this differ from the medical diagnosis? The medical diagnosis identifies the patient's disease state or the pathology and indicates a course of treatment for that state. In other words, the medical diagnosis directs the medical acts to be performed, and the nursing diagnosis directs the nursing acts to be performed. They may be treating the same basic problem, but each has a different course of action.

Are *all* patient problems amenable to nursing intervention? No, some may be more amenable to the interventions of one health-team member than another, and many problems require the combined intervention of many members. Likewise, all nursing problems are not patient problems. For example, accurate regulation of the flow of an intravenous solution is a nursing problem but not a patient problem.

The nursing diagnosis identifies that set of patient problems amenable to nursing intervention. See Figure 1.

Activities

1. Check which of the following patient problems would be amenable to nursing intervention:
   ____a. car was stolen
   ____b. fever
   ____c. loss of job
   ____d. grief over death of spouse
   ____e. impaired circulation

---

[8] *Webster's New World Dictionary of the American Language,* 1973.
[9] Gebbie, K. and Lavin, M. A., "Classifying nursing diagnoses," 1974.

© 1977 Wiley

130 NURSING ASSESSMENT

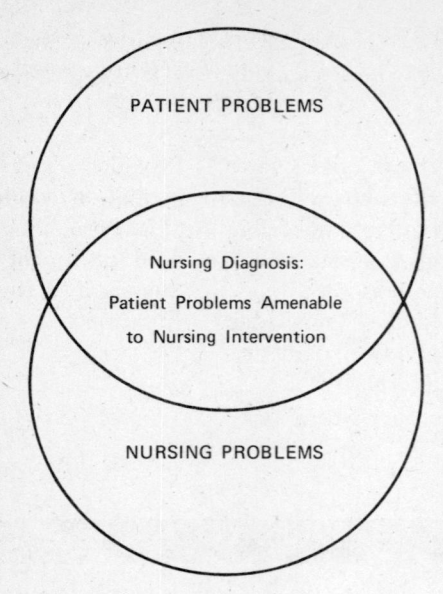

FIGURE 1
Nursing diagnosis

2. Ann works every night until 1 A.M. washing dishes in a restaurant. She has an 8 A.M. class on Monday, Wednesday, and Friday. She finds her grades are slipping, she is irritable with her friends, and she is becoming more forgetful.
   a. What are Ann's problems as they exist in this situation?
   b. Why are they occurring?
   c. Identify the relationship between your answers in a and b.
   d. Restate the definition of a problem.
   e. What are the threatened need(s)?
   f. What is the relationship of the threatened needs (e.) to the problem (a.) and the cause (b.)?

3. Ann relates her problem to Susan, a friend of hers who is a nursing student. Together they discuss the situation, determine the problem, and plan a solution.
   a. What is Susan's role in this instance?
   b. Relate this to the problem, its cause, and the unmet needs.
   c. What solution would you suggest?

ANSWERS

1. _____ a. car was stolen
   _X_ b. fever
   _____ c. loss of job
   _X_ d. grief over death of spouse
   _X_ e. impaired circulation

   Items a and b are problems, but as stated they are not health problems requiring nursing intervention. If the person needed help, the nurse could refer the person to other sources of assistance. It is conceivable that either of these could eventually lead to a health problem and require nursing intervention.

2. a. Ann's problems are: slipping grades, irritability with her friends, and becoming more forgetful.
   b. They are occurring because she is not getting sufficient sleep and rest.
   c. b (lack of sufficient sleep and rest) is the cause of a.
   d. A problem is anything that interferes or threatens to interfere with the patient's satisfaction and regulation of his needs.

© 1977 Wiley

e. The threatened needs are Ann's needs to maintain good grades (esteem needs), to maintain good relations with her friends (love or belonging needs), and to maintain her memory functions (safety or security needs).

f. Cause ⟶ Problem ⟶ Unmet neet
(b) ⟶ (a) ⟶ (e)

3. a. Ann wants to discuss her problem with someone who will help her to make a decision and then give her support in following through on her decision. Susan fulfills this role, which is one form of nursing intervention (guiding and supporting).

b. Nursing intervention's goal is to eliminate, modify, or prevent a problem so the needs can be met.

Intervention ⟶ Cause ⟶ Problem ⟶ Needs fulfilled

c. One solution might be to talk to her employer to see if her hours can be changed.

SUMMARY OF PROGRESS

At this point needs, patient problems, nursing intervention, and nursing diagnosis have been described. You have been able to identify needs, patient problems, nursing interventions, and their relationships. Next you will learn to coordinate this information to produce nursing diagnoses.

Steps in Making the Nursing Diagnosis

COLLECTION OF DATA

How do you arrive at the nursing diagnosis? The first step is the collection of data about the individual, family, or community. These data will consist of information about the health status, which in turn reflects the physiological and psychosocial state. Included will be descriptions of how the client is meeting his basic needs, of all the factors previously stated that affect the basic needs, and of how the client adapts or copes with changes in the environment. This information is sifted and analyzed for the presence of problems.

IDENTIFICATION OF PROBLEMS

Problems may be identified as either actual or potential. *Actual problems* exist and are operative in the situation, producing a difficulty or deficit in meeting a need. These may be identified by observation or by facts concerning the patient and his behavior. They may be stated as signs, symptoms, or a set of existing conditions.

Examples of actual patient problems are:

a. shortness of breath
b. malnutrition
c. pain
d. diarrhea
e. obesity
f. inappropriate affect
g. aggressive behavior
h. difficulty coping with reality of having cancer
i. inability to perform activities of daily living
j. cardiac arrest

Problems may also be *potential* in that they do not actually exist but they may develop. These are problems that are anticipated with certain diseases or conditions. The condition itself produces in the patient a lack, deficit, or inability to perform some necessary activity.

Examples of potential problems are:

a. potential shock due to hemorrhage
b. potential pulmonary complications due to inability and reluctance to cough and deep-breathe following chest surgery
c. potential skin breakdown due to immobility

© 1977 Wiley

d. potential depression secondary to diagnosis of cancer
e. potential wound infection secondary to compound fracture of tibia
f. potential difficulty giving own insulin due to poor understanding and retention of instructions about diabetes mellitus

QUALITY OF THE NURSING DIAGNOSIS

What are the criteria for a good nursing diagnosis? What are its functions? The diagnosis serves as a guide to the nurse for planning intervention. The well-stated diagnosis is a summary statement that identifies the patient problem and its cause—for example, "loss of weight due to poor dietary habits," in which loss of weight is the problem and poor dietary habits is the cause.

Activities

1. Which of the following are true statements? (Circle T or F)
    T F 1. Actual problems produce behavioral changes in the patient.
    T F 2. Potential problems would not require any nursing intervention.
    T F 3. Information leading to the diagnosis of an actual problem may be obtained from informants other than the patient.
    T F 4. Potential problems are anticipated problems.
    T F 5. Lack of knowledge about breastfeeding may be a potential problem for a pregnant woman but an actual problem for the mother of a newborn infant.

2. Check the statements that contain both a problem and its related cause:
    ___1. potential skin breakdown due to immobility
    ___2. unable to perform activities of daily living
    ___3. dehydration due to vomiting
    ___4. fever
    ___5. potential aspiration due to anesthesia of throat
    ___6. anger due to inability to care for self
    ___7. headache

3. Compare the following sets of statements. Which one is better according to these criteria? Explain why.
    a. 1. Unable to perform activities of daily living
       2. Unable to perform self-care activities below the nipple line due to immobilization in a body cast

    b. 1. Anxiety due to fear of surgery
       2. Anxiety due to lack of knowledge of outcomes of surgery

THE NURSING DIAGNOSIS **133**

    c. 1. Hostility toward staff due to unknown cause
         2. Hostility toward staff due to fear related to lack of knowledge of diagnostic procedures and possible outcomes

4. The nursing diagnosis prescribes the nursing intervention. In the following examples underline the patient problem, put parentheses around the related cause, and state the indicated nursing intervention. Compare your answers to those given below.
   a. Feelings of worthlessness due to inability to care for self because of crippling arthritis
      Nursing intervention:

   b. Fear of suffocation due to having a tracheotomy
      Nursing intervention:

   c. Pain due to myocardial infarct
      Nursing intervention:

ANSWERS
1. They are all true except number 2—potential problems do require nursing intervention.
2. You should not have checked numbers 2, 4, and 7. Why? Revise the statements. Number 2 states the problem but omits the related cause. Your revised statement may be: "Unable to

© 1977 Wiley

perform activities of daily living due to immobilization in a body cast." Numbers 4 and 7 both give only one part of the statement, and you are unsure if they are the problem or the cause. For instance, number 4, fever, may be written: "Fever due to dehydration," or, "Delirious due to fever." In the first case fever is the problem and in the second case the cause. Number 7 is the same. Headache may be the problem, as in "Headache due to anxiety," or the cause, as in "Unable to concentrate due to headache."

Further, the nursing diagnosis should be specific, clear, and patient-centered. From the statement of the problem and its cause we can derive the unmet needs, determine the goals of nursing intervention, and identify the expected outcomes in terms of the patient. In summary, a well-stated nursing diagnosis directs the nursing plan of care.

3. a. Both statements indicate the problem: the patient cannot independently meet his need to care for himself. However, the second statement is more specific: it relates the cause of this impaired ability, and it indicates that the patient can perform some activities for himself. The nurse knows that her actions will be to do for the patient what he cannot do while encouraging his independence in all other ways.
   b. Both statements indicate anxiety as the patient problem, but again the second one is a more specific guide; nursing action can provide the patient with information and thus reduce his anxiety.
   c. The second statement clearly identifies the cause of the patient's hostility. The nurse will provide the patient with information and explore the outcomes with him, thus reducing his fear and returning him to a more steady pleasant state, which is his unmet need.

4. a. *Feelings of worthlessness* (due to inability to care for self because of crippling arthritis).
   Nursing intervention: The desired outcome in this situation is that the patient's feelings of worthlessness are decreased and that he has a better self-concept. How can the nurse help to achieve that goal? If he is unable to care for himself, what other ability does he have that can be capitalized upon? Can the pain and stiffness of the arthritis be relieved so that the patient can perform limited self care? These will guide her acts of intervention.
   b. *Fear of suffocation* (due to having a tracheotomy)
   Nursing intervention: The expected outcome will be to relieve the patient of his fear of suffocation; to do so, nursing actions must be directed to explaining the purpose and nature of the tracheotomy. Actions must also instill a sense of confidence and trust in the patient that the nurse is present to support him when needed.
   c. *Pain* (due to myocardial infarct)
   Nursing intervention: The desired outcome is relief of the pain. Nursing actions will be planned taking into account the following specific knowledge the nurse has about a myocardial infarct: chest pain is due to lack of adequate blood supply, hence lack of oxygen and nutrients to the heart muscle; anxiety may be contributing to the pain; and activity may be causing an added strain and workload to the heart.

PROGRESS CHECK

So far you are doing fine. Successful completion of this module will add to your self-esteem, aid you in becoming a professional nurse, and so help fulfill your need for self-actualization. Now analyze the following situations and make the nursing diagnoses.

Situation 1. Mr. B. has been admitted to the hospital with congestive heart failure. He is 73 years old, his wife recently died, and he also has emphysema and arthritis. He declines to eat, cries a lot, is forgetful, and states that he is "not good for anything."

© 1977 Wiley

THE NURSING DIAGNOSIS **135**

Situation 2. Tom has had chest surgery for removal of a tumor. You have observed that he remains in the same position for long periods, that his breathing is shallow, that he is not coughing, and that he winces when he does move.

Situation 3. Mrs. S. is in the surgical intensive care unit after being struck by a car. She has a tracheostomy for breathing, her pelvis is fractured, she is immobilized in traction, and she is receiving intravenous therapy in both arms. She is conscious but unable to speak or move because of the apparatus. She moves her head slightly, taking in her surroundings, there is a look of fear on her face, and she begins to cry.

Situation 4. Ann Chu has come to the doctor complaining of sore throat, fever, runny nose, and general discomfort. The doctor diagnoses her condition as a severe cold and prescribes that she take aspirin 10 gr every 4 hours for elevated temperature, force fluids, and restrict her activity. She is 16 years old, of Vietnamese origin, and just newly arrived in this country.

ANSWERS
Situation 1. Mr. B has experienced the loss of his wife and he is also physically incapacitated, another form of loss. His responses are typical symptoms of depression, so you could summarize the situation with the following nursing diagnosis:

Depression and grief due to loss of wife and loss of his own physical abilities.

Situation 2. Shallow breathing and lack of coughing postsurgically should indicate to you the potential development of respiratory complications such as atelectasis. You also notice that he is not moving and that he winces when he moves, which postsurgically is probably caused by pain, which you can validate with him. Your nursing diagnosis is:
1. pain secondary to chest surgery
2. potential for respiratory complications due to inadequate ventilation due to pain, incision, and trauma of chest surgery

Situation 3. The behavior you observe is fear and crying. All of the factors could be causing the fear, but the patient cannot communicate the exact cause or discuss her fears. She is confined and immobilized, so that she cannot do anything. Her nursing diagnosis might be:

Fear, powerlessness due to inability to perform any act by herself or to communicate. (There will also be other nursing diagnoses in this situation related to actual and potential physiological problems.)

Situation 4. You might ask: what problem does she have that requires nursing intervention? Consider that she is from a different culture and she may not understand the doc-

© 1977 Wiley

tor's instructions. What exactly do "force fluids" and "restrict activity" mean? Also consider her stage of development—a teenager: often they do not realize the need to follow a medical regimen. Analyzing this, her nursing diagnosis might be:

Potential for nonadherence to medical therapy due to lack of understanding of importance of doctor's prescription.

POSTTEST

You should be able to complete the posttest with 100% mastery. If you do not, review any of the parts in this module that caused you difficulty.

A. Fill-in-the-blanks (Fill in the words to complete the following sentences)
1. Something that is required is a/n _____. If there is any form of interference in supplying this requirement, then a _____ exists. The nurse who recognizes this interference will evaluate the situation from available data and make a _____. From this she will plan her _____.

B. Multiple-choice (Circle the letter of the one best answer)
2. Which of the following statements describe patient problems?
    1. Doctors treat all patient problems.
    2. They are health problems.
    3. They reflect imbalance in physiological and psychosocial need satisfaction.
    4. Nurses treat all patient problems.
        a. 1, 2
        b. 2, 3
        c. 2, 3, 4
        d. all of the above

3. Which of the following statements apply to the description of needs?
    1. They are necessities.
    2. They are influenced by health status, social status, and developmental status.
    3. They vary from day to day.
    4. They must be completely satisfied for man to exist.
        a. 1, 2
        b. 2, 3
        c. 1, 2, 4
        d. all except 4

4. According to its definition, which of the following are examples of nursing intervention?
    1. giving instructions in taking insulin
    2. telling the doctor about an elevated temperature
    3. assigning the more experienced R.N.'s to the more difficult patients
    4. reducing the noise in the intensive care unit
        a. 1, 2, 4
        b. 1, 4
        c. 2, 3
        d. all of the above

5. According to its definition, which of the following is/are statement(s) of nursing diagnosis?
    1. headaches, increased blood pressure, with anxiety

© 1977 Wiley

2. respiratory insufficiency
3. infertility
4. loneliness due to loss of spouse
    a. 1, 4
    b. 2, 3
    c. 4 only
    d. all of the above

6. Arrange the following in the sequential order of steps for making a nursing diagnosis:
    1. identify unmet needs.
    2. analyze observations, facts.
    3. collect data base.
    4. formulate summary statement.
    5. relate to realm of nursing.
        a. 3, 2, 1, 5, 4
        b. 3, 1, 2, 4, 5
        c. 2, 3, 1, 4, 5
        d. 1, 2, 3, 5, 4

7. Which of the following statements describe potential patient problems?
    1. They do not require nursing intervention.
    2. They are observable in the patient.
    3. They are anticipated.
    4. They are derived from existing disease conditions.
        a. 1, 3
        b. 2, 4
        c. 2, 3
        d. 3, 4

8. The lack of a stated cause in the nursing diagnosis will create the greatest difficulty in:
    a. defining the expected outcomes of care
    b. determining the unmet need
    c. focusing the attention of nursing intervention
    d. identifying the problem

9. What main purpose does the following nursing diagnosis serve?
   Obesity due to lack of sufficient exercise and overeating
    a. identifies obesity as the problem
    b. identifies lack of sufficient exercise and overeating as a cause
    c. indicates patient has an unmet need to have desirable weight
    d. directs plan of care to achieve loss of weight

10. "Situations that threaten an individual's self-concept will cause anxiety."
    In this statement which of the following relationships are true?
    a. anxiety is the problem causing threatened self-concept
    b. threatened self-concept is the problem causing anxiety
    c. self-concept is the need that is threatened
    d. both b and c are true
    How would you state this as a nursing diagnosis?

11. Which of the following nursing interventions would be most effective in the above situation?
    a. actions to eliminate the situation
    b. actions to decrease the anxiety
    c. compliments to improve the individual's self-concept
    d. actions to decrease the individual's sensitivity to his needs

© 1977 Wiley

138 NURSING ASSESSMENT

C. **Matching** In the following list put N in front of examples of a Need and P in front of examples of a Patient Problem.
   ____1. self-respect
   ____2. infertility
   ____3. respiratory insufficiency
   ____4. increased blood pressure
   ____5. evaluation of self
   ____6. orientation
   ____7. involvement in care
   ____8. inability to stand

D. **Compare and Evaluate** The statements below are grouped in threes. Using the criteria for a well-stated nursing diagnosis, compare and evaluate the statements within each group.
   1. impairment of verbal communication due to fractured mandible
   2. rash
   3. inadequate resources for medical care due to living in deprived area

   4. shortness of breath
   5. needs assistance with eating
   6. refuses to comply with treatment

   7. needs instruction in how to treat burn
   8. potential impaired nutritional state secondary to gastrointestinal surgery
   9. arthritis

E. **Analyze the following situations**
   a. Summarize the data into a well-stated nursing diagnosis.
   b. State the indicated nursing intervention and the goals in terms of patient outcomes.

© 1977 Wiley

Situation 1: Mr. Brown has a history of peptic ulcer. For two days he has been having tarry stools that are positive for blood. During patient rounds you observe that he is pale, perspiring, and appears apprehensive. You take his vital signs and find blood pressure 90/60 and pulse 120.

Situation 2: A 60-year-old man with a fractured hip is your patient and he is in traction. He says he doesn't want to be a bother to the nurses. He tries to pour himself a drink and spills water in the bed. During the night he knocks his urinal off the bedside stand and is discovered trying to undo his traction "so he can clean up the mess."

Answers

A. **Fill in the blanks**
   1. need, problem, nursing diagnosis, nursing intervention

B. **Multiple choice**
   2. b 3. d 4. a 5. c 6. a 7. d 8. c 9. d 10. d;
   Anxiety due to threatened self-concept due to (provoking) situations. 11. a

C. **Matching**
   1. N 2. P 3. P 4. P 5. N 6. N 7. N 8. P

D. **Compare and Evaluate**
   1, 2, 3:
   Statements 1 and 3 both have a problem and cause. Statement 2, rash, is an incomplete statement—probably a problem, although it may be a cause of something, such as itching. Statement 1 is more amenable to nursing intervention. Statement 3 may require the help of a social worker.

© 1977 Wiley

4, 5, 6:

None of these is an adequate statement. Statement 4, shortness of breath, is a problem, but unless one knows its cause there is no focus for nursing action. Statement 5, needs assistance with eating, is neither problem nor cause. Remember: a problem is a difficulty or interference, and the fact that "the patient needs so-and-so" is not the problem. Statement 6, refuses to comply with treatment, is also incomplete, and we cannot tell whether it is a problem or cause of a problem.

7, 8, 9:

Statement 8 is adequate, giving both a potential problem and its related cause. It directs the nurse to observe the patient for signs of impaired nutritional state (fluid and electrolyte imbalance, weakness, nervous system changes, etc.) and to take actions to avoid these. Statement 7, like 5, states a need. Statement 9, arthritis, is incomplete. It indicates the pathology but does not state what problem is arising from the arthritis that is treatable by nursing intervention. More focus is needed—the problem may be pain, limited motion, despondency, etc.

E. **Analysis of situations**

Situation 1:
a. *Nursing diagnosis.* Potential hemorrhage due to peptic ulcer.
b. *Nursing intervention and patient outcome.* The problem is potential hemorrhage, which threatens Mr. Brown's physiological safety. Nursing intervention will be directed to the cause, peptic ulcer. Activities would include observation and reporting of signs and symptoms and support of the medical regimen. The expected patient outcome would be no hemorrhage.

Situation 2:
a. *Nursing diagnosis.* Anxiety due to threatened self-concept due to inability to care for self due to being immobilized by traction for fractured hip.
b. *Nursing intervention and patient outcome.* The problem is anxiety, which is interfering with this man's need to maintain his self-concept. Nursing intervention will be directed to the cause, inability to care for self. Nursing activities would include giving the man as much independence as possible in caring for himself, providing some activity for him that would be useful and productive (sorting the mail, stamping forms), and praising him for his efforts. The expected patient outcome would be decreased anxiety with removal of the threat to his self-concept.

References

Bower, Fay Louise, *The Process of Planning Nursing Care: A Theoretical Model.* St. Louis: C. V. Mosby, 1972, p. 68.

Gebbie, K. and Lavin, M. A., "Classifying nursing diagnoses," *American Journal of Nursing,* 4 (1974): 250–253.

Maslow, A. H., *Motivation and Personality.* New York: Harper & Row, 1954.

Webster's New World Dictionary of the American Language. Cleveland: The World Publishing Co., 1973, pp. 163, 304, 383.

Suggested Reading

Becknell, E. P., and Smith, D. M., *System of Nursing Practice.* Philadelphia: F. A. Davis, 1975.

Bloch, D., "Some crucial terms in nursing, what do they really mean?" *Nursing Outlook* 22 (1974): 689–694.

Johnson, M. M.; Davis, M. C.; and Bilitch, J. J., *Problem-Solving in Nursing Practice.* Dubuque, Iowa: Wm. C. Brown, 1970.

Mayers, M. G., *A Systematic Approach to the Nursing Care Plan.* New York: Appleton-Century-Crofts, 1972.

Monken, S. S., "After assessment—what then?," *Nursing Clinics of North America* 10 (1975): 107–120.

Mundinger, M. O. and Jauron, G. D., "Developing a nursing diagnosis," *Nursing Outlook,* 23 (1975): 94–98.

Roy, C., Sr., "A diagnostic classification system for nursing," *Nursing Outlook,* 23 (1975): 90–94.

Yura, H. and Walsh, M. B., *The Nursing Process,* 2nd ed. New York: Appleton-Century-Crofts, 1973.

SUZANNE HALL JOHNSON, R.N., M.N.

WILEY NURSING CONCEPT MODULE

THE EVALUATION PROCESS

CONTENTS

    PRETEST 145   Answers 146

    INTRODUCTION 147

    TERMINAL OBJECTIVES 147

        ACTIVITY 1.   The Evaluation Process   148
            Part A: Usefulness of Evaluation in Nursing   148
            Part B: Evaluation as Part of the Problem-Solving Process   153
        ACTIVITY 2.   Evaluation Criteria   155
        ACTIVITY 3.   Actions in the Evaluation Process   160
        ACTIVITY 4.   Planning and Performing the Evaluation   163

    POSTTEST 164   Answers 166

    REFERENCES 166

    SUGGESTED READINGS 167

© 1977 Wiley

PRETEST

Complete the following questions in the spaces provided.

1. Complete the blanks in the following definition of evaluation process. The evaluation process is a group of related _____ that rate a _____ based on specific _____.

The following statements concern characteristics or values of the evaluation process. Answer each statement as True or False.

T F 2. The evaluation process is concerned only with past performances.

T F 3. The main value of the evaluation process is its punitive function to nurses who are not meeting the standards of practice.

T F 4. The evaluation process is an independent part of the problem-solving process.

T F 5. The evaluation process begins along with the assessment part of problem solving.

T F 6. Consumers independently set up standards to evaluate health care.

T F 7. Nursing care is adequately evaluated with the use of interdisciplinary medical criteria.

T F 8. Peer evaluation is often more precise than supervisor evaluation.

T F 9. Previous knowledge of the performance criteria usually increases the nurse's fear before an evaluation conference.

10. List three benefits you might receive from a supervisor's evaluation of your nursing performance.
    a.
    b.
    c.

Three types of evaluation for the health team are listed below. Mark the characteristic that best describes each type of evaluation in the space provided.

____ 11. utilization review   a. evaluates a client's health care through chart review
____ 12. quality assurance   b. evaluates the use of health personnel
____ 13. patient care audit   c. determines whether a group of clients meet the desired outcome criteria

A list of evaluation criteria is provided below. Each criterion has at least one essential characteristic missing. State the missing characteristic and rewrite each criterion to include that element.

14. Criterion: Following surgery the client exercised for a half hour each day.
    Missing characteristic:
    Revised criterion:

15. Criterion: The client's blood pressure was between 140 to 160 systolic and 80 to 95 diastolic within four hours of the initiation of anti-hypertensive medication.
    Missing characteristic:
    Revised criterion:

16. The client initiated verbal conversation with at least two other people in the day room.
    Missing characteristic:
    Revised criterion:

© 1977 Wiley

145

146 NURSING ASSESSMENT

Demonstrate the planning and performance of the evaluation process by answering the questions on the clinical situation below. This evaluation will focus on the nurse.

Situation: As a new nurse in a cardiac care unit you recognize that you cannot read the electrocardiograms to describe specific arrhythmias.

17. *Assessment:* Describe what abilities and needs you have in this situation.

18. *Goals:* Identify one nurse goal related to this situation.

19. *Criterion:* Develop one process criterion for the nursing actions.

Situation: You have completed a course in electrocardiogram interpretation. You passed the test by identifying five of the five types of arrhythmias on the test. Since the course you have correctly identified four of the six arrhythmias you have seen on the cardiac unit.

20. *Comparison:* Using the additional information above, compare the result of the nursing action with the process criteria.

GOOD! You have completed the Pretest. Check the answers to determine your score in the Pretest. Each question is worth one point. You must have seventeen points (85%) correct to pass the Pretest.

Answers

1. actions, performance, criteria
2. F   3. F   4. F   5. T   6. T   7. F   8. T   9. F
10. increased self-worth, continued learning, increased stature or position, passing promotion or pay increase, increased quality of nursing performance (any three)
11. b. utilization review—evaluates the use of health personnel
12. c. quality assurance—determines whether a group of clients meet the desired outcome criteria
13. a. patient care audit—evaluates a client's health care through chart review
14. not observable (example of a revised criterion: "following surgery the client raised both arms above the head fifteen times in ½ hour per day")
15. not single (example revised criterion: "the client's blood pressure was between 140 to 160 systolic following . . .")
16. not timed (example revised criterion: "one week after the nurse started a plan to reward the client for each verbal contact, he initiated verbal conversation with at least two other people per day")
17. *Assessment:* unable to read electrocardiograms
18. *Goal:* be able to identify arrhythmias on electrocardiograms
19. *Criterion:* any criterion that evaluates the nurse's actions and is critical, single, observable, timed, and positive (example: "the nurse will identify correctly five out of five irregular patterns she observed on the unit following an electrocardiogram course")
20. Answer will depend on the criterion selected above. The nurse meets the criterion if five of five in the course is used or four of six on the unit. Does not meet criterion above.

© 1977 Wiley

THE EVALUATION PROCESS **147**

INTRODUCTION

This module presents the major components of the evaluation process in nursing. It emphasizes the formation and utilization of specific evaluation criteria. By the end of the module the reader will be able to develop and use specific evaluation criteria to evaluate nursing care.

Directions

1. Determine what is required of you and its value to you by reading the introduction and objectives.
2. Identify your background abilities in evaluation by completing the prerequisite section.
3. Follow the directions in Activities 1, 2, and 3 which require you to apply the concepts of evaluation to your clinical experiences.
4. After finishing all the activities, determine if you have successfully met the objectives by completing the Posttest.

Prerequisites

This module builds on your knowledge and skill in problem solving. Answer each question below to determine your background in the problem-solving process.

1. When you assess a client, do you describe specific characteristics or actions?   Yes   No
2. When you describe a client's problem, do you base it on precise data from your assessment?   Yes   No
3. When you plan interventions, do you consider many types of action that might reduce the problem?   Yes   No

If you answered Yes to the questions above, you have the basic concepts in the problem-solving process that are prerequisites for this module; please continue in this module.

If you answered No to any of the questions above, you have not mastered these concepts in problem solving. Review the components of the problem-solving process in any text on the nursing process. When you have mastered these concepts, continue in this module.

TERMINAL OBJECTIVES

By the end of the module the reader will:

1. define "evaluation process"
2. predict the value of the evaluation process
3. identify the characteristics of different types of evaluation for groups
4. differentiate between process and outcome evaluation criteria
5. determine the relationship between the evaluation process and the problem-solving process
6. analyze and develop evaluation criteria based on specific criteria
7. analyze a clinical situation to design, organize, and demonstrate the evaluation of nursing care

© 1977 Wiley

148 NURSING ASSESSMENT

ACTIVITY 1
THE EVALUATION PROCESS

Activity 1 describes the use of evaluation, defines the word evaluation, introduces the trends affecting evaluation today, and describes the relationship between the evaluation process and the problem-solving process.

Part A: Usefulness of Evaluation in Nursing

PAST EXPERIENCES WITH EVALUATION
When the word "evaluation" is mentioned, most people think of the tests they took in school or of ratings by a supervisor. Nurses often picture the clinical course evaluation by the instructor, the nurse licensure examination by the state, or the staff nurse competence rating by the supervisor.

In all the evaluation situations above, the evaluation is being performed by a person who has great authority over the nurse's professional or financial goal. These are situations of high anxiety and feelings of threatened self-worth for the nurse.

Questions:
1. a. Describe one situation when you were evaluated.

   b. Who was the person who did the evaluation?

   c. Did this person have great authority over you?

POSITIVE EVALUATION
Many of a nurse's uses of evaluation can result in positive feelings. A nurse who evaluates nursing care by observing the performance of the dressing change and comparing it to criteria of sterile technique supports satisfactory performance and builds feelings of self-worth.

Questions:
2. a. Describe one situation when you observed your own nursing performance.

   b. Did you feel positive about your accomplishment?

WAYS TO MAKE EVALUATION POSITIVE
Evaluation is positive when it is used as a method of feedback that supports your accomplishments and guides your progress. The key to positive experiences in evaluation is to set up a method of

© 1977 Wiley

ongoing self-evaluation by:

1. defining what is expected
2. planning and participating in activities to develop the expected performance
3. seeking feedback and ongoing evaluation to guide the performance as it develops

This positive self-evaluation not only helps you meet the expectations; it allows you to feel excited about accomplishing them. Evaluation in this form supports the nurse's self-worth.

For example, Janie, a student nurse, has done satisfactory work in her clinical courses; however, she is very nervous and fearful on every evaluation day. If she (1) sought out the teacher and course expectations, (2) set up experiences to refine her performance in weak areas, and (3) sought feedback from patients, nurses, and instructor as she developed, she would know how well she was doing and she could feel confident in her evaluation.

Questions:
3. a. Describe one clinical nursing skill you need to develop or refine.

   b. List one experience that would help you refine your performance in this area.

   c. Briefly describe how you could get client, staff, or teacher feedback before the critical evaluation day.

   d. Would this self-evaluation help you refine your nursing care?

   e. Would this self-evaluation support your feelings of self-worth?

DEFINITION OF THE EVALUATION PROCESS
The evaluation process is a group of related *actions* that rate a *performance* based on specific *criteria*. The goal of evaluation is not only to determine if a performance meets the criteria but to stimulate the attainment of that performance.

Question:
4. State the definition of evaluation process in your own words.

BENEFITS OF THE EVALUATION PROCESS
The many benefits of the evaluation process for the nurse include:

1. feelings of self-worth and confidence due to knowledge of meeting criteria of successful performance

© 1977 Wiley

150 NURSING ASSESSMENT

2. continued learning due to knowledge of not meeting criteria
3. increased stature or position due to the ability to describe to another professional what the nurse does and the beneficial outcomes
4. a passing promotion or pay increase due to the ability to describe the nurse's performance and the beneficial results to a teacher, supervisor, or administrator
5. development of quality nursing care due to a process that compares the actual nursing care to optimal care

Question:
5. List at least three benefits you would get from performing a self-evaluation of your clinical practice.

FUTURE DEMANDS FOR NURSING EVALUATION

As mentioned, the most common methods of evaluation in nursing are the instructor or supervisor rating by means of a test or a list of performance criteria. There are additional demands on nursing to develop more evaluation methods. Three present trends are making evaluation even more important to nurses.

One trend is the increased cost of health care, which results in the health administrator's close scrutiny of cost and benefit. The administrator wants to know that the nurse is performing the nursing role for the salary the hospital is paying. Therefore, specific performance standards and other methods of evaluating staff are being developed.

Second, the consumer's demand for equal rights in health care has increased the consumer's participation in the evaluation of health care. Health care functions to promote the consumer's health; the consumer must be considered in the evaluation of the effectiveness of that care.

Third, large amounts of local, state, and federal money are going to health care. To determine that this money is utilized to provide the best quantity and quality of care, a method of health-care evaluation must be developed in health agencies. Local, state, and federal laws have been passed that require an evaluation of the effectiveness of health care.

Several types of evaluation methods have been developed to evaluate the health care of large groups of people.

1. utilization review evaluates the extent of use of health facilities and manpower.[1,2]
2. quality assurance includes an evaluation of the quality of health care given.[3]
3. patient care audit is most commonly a retrospective review of the nursing action and patient outcomes during an illness.[4]

Utilization review, quality assurance, and the patient care audit are three types of evaluation used to determine the effective or efficient use of health-care facilities and personnel. These systems for the evaluation of health care provided groups of people are based on the evaluation process described in this module.

Review processes such as the ones above are rapidly being developed. Nurses must participate in the formation of the evaluation methods. Nurses will help form evaluation criteria that take account of the clients', families', and communities' views of health. They will help determine the significance of health care by forming criteria to evaluate the effectiveness of health teaching and home care.

[1] McClain, J. O., "Screening for Utilization Review," 1973.
[2] Tippett, J., "Developing a Utilization Review Model for Community Medical Health Centers," 1975.
[3] Maniaci, Marie, "Quality Assurance in the Provision of Hospital Care: Case Study," 1974.
[4] Eddy, Lyndall and Westbrook, Linda, "Multidisciplinary Retrospective Patient Care Audit," 1975.

© 1977 Wiley

Questions:
6. a. Would you rather participate in developing criteria to evaluate your nursing performance or have the state establish the criteria that evaluate your care?

   b. Describe the terms *utilization review, quality assurance,* and *patient care audit.*

NURSES' ROLE IN EVALUATION

Pressures from health administrators, consumers, and public organizations are forcing the development of new methods for the evaluation of health care. Nurses must evaluate and support their performance in the provision of health care.[5] They must develop and identify actions that are beneficial in promoting health care for the client. Only after nurses demonstrates their significant role in promoting health will the public value their role and provide financial rewards.

Questions:
7. a. List one intervention you have performed that promoted health in a client.

   b. How could you describe the value of your action to another person?

STAFF AND PEER EVALUATION

In addition to the above trends the decentralization of authority has placed more decisions in the role of the staff nurse. Now self-evaluations and peer evaluations are being instituted in schools and health centers.[6] The trend is supported by the fact that the closest observer to your performance is you and the next closest is your peer.

An evaluation that describes an individual's exact performance compared to stated criteria is very powerful in supporting or motivating the individual. The individual and his coworkers have the best opportunity to describe continuous specific behaviors, therefore, self and peer evaluations are very valuable.

---

[5] Orme, J. V., "Nurse Participation in Medical Peer Review," 1974.
[6] Gold, H. et al., "Peer Review, A Working Experience," 1973.

Questions:
8. a. From your last clinical practice, describe one nursing intervention you performed.

Evaluate your own performance by answering the questions below.
   b. Did you perform this action according to guidelines for that skill?

   c. Did the desired outcome or expected client change occur from your action?

SUMMARY
It is important for a nurse to participate in evaluations of self, peers, nursing care, and health care. Evaluation of any number of people or types of performance is based on a common evaluation process, which is presented in subsequent Activities in the module.

CONGRATULATIONS! You have completed Part A of Activity 1. Please go on to the answers below. When you have answered the questions correctly and reviewed them for any wrong answers, proceed to Part B.

Answers

1. a. any evaluation experience
    b. usually a supervisor or teacher, but any evaluator is acceptable
    c. usually the evaluator will have great authority
2. a. description of any nursing experience
    b. feeling of positive or negative achievement related to the nursing experience described in item a
3. a. description of any clinical nursing skill
    b. any experience that would develop the skill in item a
    c. description of interaction with client, staff, or teacher for feedback on nursing skill
    d. yes, evaluating present abilities and weaknesses would help continued refinement of nursing care.
    e. yes, if the evaluation shows the performance met the criteria; no, if the evaluation shows the performance did not meet the criteria.
4. A definition of evaluation that stresses *actions*, that looks at *performance*, and that utilizes *criteria*.
5. Three individual benefits similar to (1) increased self-worth, (2) continued learning, (3) increased stature or position, (4) passed promotion or pay increase, and (5) increased quality of nursing care.
6. a. rather help set up criteria to evaluate nursing than have the state set them up
    b. see the Activity for characteristics of the group evaluation methods
7. a. one nursing action that has promoted health in a client
    b. description of the beneficial effects on the patient resulting from the nursing action described in item a

© 1977 Wiley

8. a. one nursing intervention performed in clinical practice
    b. yes, if the action was performed on the guidelines; no, if not
    c. yes, if the desired client change occurred; no, if not

Part B: Evaluation as Part of The Problem-Solving Process

The problem-solving process is basically that of identifying a problem (assessment), describing the problem (problem statement), deciding on a performance activity (intervention), and determining that the problem has been solved (evaluation).

Evaluation is an essential element which, if omitted, prevents the problem-solving process from being successful. The process is successful if the problem is solved; we cannot determine this without an evaluation.

An evaluation is needed to determine the success of a nursing action. When a mother comes to clinic with a three-month-old infant, the nurse assesses the infant for the normal weight and height and for normal behaviors. The nurse who identifies a mother's fear that something the baby is doing is abnormal often "reassures" the mother that the baby is "normal" and "do not worry." The nurse often fails to evaluate the success of her measures by evaluating the changes in the mother's fears. Sometimes the "reassurance" only produces more anxiety. The only way to determine if a problem is solved is to evaluate whether the desired outcome has been reached.

Questions:
1. a. Describe one incident when you identified a client's problem and performed an intervention to solve it.

    b. Did you actually evaluate the changes in the client's situation that demonstrated the problem was solved? What were the changes that showed the reduction in the problem?

    c. Is it correct to assume a client's problem is solved because you performed a usual intervention?

RELATION OF THE EVALUATION TO THE ASSESSMENT
An evaluation is closely related to the initial assessment. The essential part of a successful evaluation process (and problem-solving process) is an *assessment* that gathers data that are descriptive and specific for the client. The only way to evaluate that a characteristic is changed is to know exactly what the characteristic is before something is done to change it. An evaluation that is based on the initial specific assessment describes the change in the characteristic for that client.

© 1977 Wiley

For example: A nurse assesses that a pregnant adolescent client averages two glasses of milk a day and other proteins to average 38 grams of protein each day. The nurse determines this is below that required for an adolescent pregnant woman and intervenes with a teaching program. Four weeks later this nurse will evaluate the client's average protein intake and determine if the problem of low protein has been resolved. Without the exact description of the foods or grams originally eaten the nurse would not be able to clearly evaluate the client's change.

Question:
2. Jerry Folk, a twelve-year-old boy, is admitted to your unit in status asthmaticus. You assess his respiratory wheezing, straight sitting position, and perspiration as signs of the problem of respiratory difficulty. You have positioned him with back support, asked his mother to sit by his bed quietly and hold his hand if he likes, and you have started broncho-dilator medications as ordered. What changes in Jerry's condition would show you that your interventions were successful?

RELATIONSHIP OF THE EVALUATION TO THE PROBLEM

A second component of an evaluation is that it must relate to the *problem statement*. An evaluation that is based only on the initial assessment can show only that the characteristic has changed. In order for an evaluation to determine that the problem has indeed been solved, it must evaluate the many different characteristics that are related to the problem.

For example, with the pregnant adolescent the evaluation of the number of grams of protein is only one factor in determining that she has sufficient protein intake. Another factor related to the problem of low protein intake must be evaluated. Does this client have adequate blood cell volume and is she active and energetic? These factors determine if the client has sufficient iron intake in the protein and are essential in evaluating her protein needs.

An effective evaluation includes not only a reassessment of the initial characteristics that demonstrated the problem but also other characteristics that are related to the problem.

Question:
3. In the situation of Jerry Folk, one client problem is difficulty with respirations. List at least one additional characteristic that would describe the state of his respiratory difficulty.

RELATIONSHIP OF THE EVALUATION TO THE INTERVENTION

An evaluation must also relate to the interventions instituted. Since one purpose of nursing evaluation is to determine the quality of nursing care performed, the evaluation must be related to the nursing interventions. An evaluation of nursing care must include criteria that are related not to the medical decisions and orders but to the nursing actions.

For example, Thomas, a client, has been undergoing radiation therapy after a colostomy operation for sigmoid cancer. An evaluation stating no further cancer spread would evaluate the success of the surgery and radiation but might be less related to the nursing intervention. The patient's ability to take independent steps in caring for his colostomy is more related to the nurse's actions of teaching and emotional support. Therefore, the patient's ability to care for his colostomy within two weeks is a criterion for evaluation that is related to nursing actions.

Question:
4. In Jerry's situation with respiratory difficulty the nurse directed his mother to use more touch and less discussion to help reduce his respiratory effort in talking. Describe one characteristic that would change partly due to this nursing intervention.

© 1977 Wiley

EVALUATION AS PART OF THE PROBLEM-SOLVING PROCESS

Evaluation is an essential part of the problem-solving process. The evaluation criteria are based on the assessment, problem, and intervention phases of the process.

A difficulty many nurses experience in evaluation is failure to plan the evaluation along with the assessment, problem, and interventions. An effective evaluation cannot be performed only after an action is taken. Once the action has occurred, you have lost the initial characteristic you wanted to change. Without planning for evaluation in the assessment phases, the nurse cannot show how the actions were helpful, because she cannot describe the changes.

Question:
5. What components of the nursing practice are used to plan an effective evaluation?

NICE! You have now completed Part B of Activity 1. Compare your answers with those that follow, and return to the section to review any material necessary. After you have answered all the questions successfully, you have completed Activity 1. Please go to Activity 2.

Answers
1. a. any clinical incident resulting in identification of a client's problem
   b. yes, for an evaluation of the client's changes after your intervention; no, if you did not evaluate the client's changes after intervention
   c. no; to determine if a client's problem is solved you must determine the changes in the client
2. reduced respiratory wheezing, lying flat in bed, dry skin
3. blood oxygen level, skin color, respiratory and cardiac rate, respiratory volume, activity such as working or talking and many other characteristics related to respiratory effort
4. characteristics such as: Jerry would hold his mother's hand, Jerry would not talk for period of at least thirty minutes
5. assessment, problem, and intervention

ACTIVITY 2

EVALUATION CRITERIA

Activity 2 describes the characteristics of any evaluation criteria and presents process and outcome types of criteria.

Forming Evaluation Criteria

EVALUATION CRITERIA

An evaluation criterion is a statement of a critical *condition* or *behavior*.[7] For example:

Example Criterion

a. Client is able to feed herself all meals by the second day following surgery.

Interpretation

a. Critical? Yes, it may be critical for many types of clients.
   Behavior? Yes.
   Critical Behavior? Yes.

---

[7] Yura, Helen, and Walsh, Mary, *Guidelines for Review of Nursing Care at the Local Level*, 1976.

© 1977 Wiley

b. Client is able to be independent by the second week after surgery.

b. Critical? Yes, may be critical for many clients.
Behavior? No. Not observable behaviors.
Critical Behavior? No.

Question:
1. What is an evaluation criterion?

EVALUATION CRITERION: THE CRITICAL BEHAVIOR OR CHARACTERISTIC
An evaluation criterion must describe a critical behavior or characteristic. Since it must show whether something meets a certain desired factor, the criterion should be:

1. critical
2. single
3. observable
4. timed
5. positive

These characteristics of the evaluation criterion will be discussed below.

CRITICAL CHARACTERISTIC OF THE CRITERION
An evaluation criterion must be of a critical nature. It must be important to the person or activity evaluated. The criterion must describe a point of exact position when a characteristic is attained.

Questions:
Identify each characteristic below as being critical or not critical for the client's problem.

2. a. Thirty-pound weight loss within six weeks for a moderately obese client. Critical?   Noncritical?
   b. Finishing reading a magazine for a client who has difficulty socializing with other people. Critical?   Noncritical?
   c. Completed knitting a blanket for her first grandchild by a client with arthritis in her hands. Critical?   Noncritical?

SINGLE CHARACTERISTIC OF THE CRITERION
It is important to have an evaluation criterion that describes a single behavior or characteristic. If two characteristics are included in one criterion, it is difficult to determine if the criterion is met if only one of the two behaviors is performed. When two behaviors are important, include each as a single criterion.

Questions:
Criterion: Loss of thirty pounds and two inches at the waist in six weeks for a moderately obese client.

3. a. Is the above criterion a single characteristic or behavior?
   b If not, rewrite the criterion to include a single characteristic.

© 1977 Wiley

OBSERVABLE CHARACTERISTIC IN THE CRITERION

It is essential for the evaluation criterion to describe an observable behavior or condition. Specific behaviors or characteristics are observable and often are even measurable by means of a rating scale or instrument.

The thirty-pound weight loss is a measurable criterion, since weight can be measured on an acceptable scale. A measurable criterion is observable to the point of being quantified.

A statement such as "the client regained his appetite" is not an observable behavior or condition. To make the criterion more measurable, the statement must be more specific, "The client drinks 1,200 cc in twenty-four hours" or "the client eats eight ounces of meat in twenty-four hours" are measurable criteria. "The client eats all of the food on his breakfast tray" is an observable criterion.

Questions:
Criterion: Independent functioning within five days following abdominal surgery for appendicitis.

4. a. Is the above criterion an observable characteristic or behavior?
   b. If not, rewrite the criterion to include an observable characteristic.

TIMED CHARACTERISTIC IN THE CRITERION

It is essential for the evaluation criterion to specify a time when the behavior should occur. For example, "voiding at least 200 cc after surgery" with no time limit would not tell you whether the client's urinary system is functioning correctly or incorrectly. "Voiding 200 cc total in the first six hours following surgery" is a timed criterion that would evaluate whether the client's urinary system was functioning correctly. Voiding of 200 cc total in the twenty-four hours following surgery does not meet the criterion and is a sign of an acute urinary or circulatory problem.

Questions:
Criterion: The client states the correct schedule for his medications.

5. a. Does the above criterion include a timed characteristic?
   b. If not, rewrite the criterion to include a timed characteristic or behavior.

POSITIVE FACTORS IN THE CRITERION

It is important for the evaluation criterion to describe a positive expected result—an actual condition. Positive criteria describe something that should occur; negative criteria describe something that should not occur.

For example, the criterion "intact skin" is a positive one describing a desired condition. The criterion "no bleeding" is a negative one describing an undesirable condition or the absence of a condition.

It is best to use positive factors in a criterion, because they describe a condition that can be observed, while negative factors describe the lack of a condition, which is difficult to substantiate.

Questions:
Criterion: No medication error.

6. a. Does the above criterion include a positive behavior?
   b. If not, rewrite the criterion in a positive form.

© 1977 Wiley

INCLUDING THE ESSENTIAL ELEMENTS IN THE EVALUATION CRITERION
In review, the evaluation criterion must describe a critical, single, observable, timed, and positive behavior or characteristic.

Questions:
Criterion: The client understands his expected postoperative care.
   Rewrite the criterion above to include all the essential elements listed below.

7. a. Include a single behavior or condition in the criterion.
   b. Include a critical behavior or condition in the criterion.
   c. Refine the criterion to include an observable behavior or condition.
   d. Include a specific time for the occurrence of the critical behavior or condition.
   e. state the behavior or condition in a positive way.

PROCESS AND OUTCOME EVALUATION CRITERIA
Although they all include the five essential elements described above, evaluation criteria can be classified into two groups, depending on whether the subject is the nurse or the client. The evaluation criteria that focus on the nurse's action are called *process* criteria; those that focus on the client outcome are called *outcome* criteria.

For a nurse who teaches the client the use of blow bottles for deep breathing, a criterion that evaluates the action is "the nurse demonstrates the deep breathing process that is expected during the teaching session." It is the nurse's action that is being evaluated, so the evaluation criterion is a *process* criterion. A criterion that evaluates the client's outcome condition is "The client blows the water from one bottle to the other following the nurse's teaching." Here the client's response to the nurse's teaching is being evaluated, so the criterion is an *outcome* criterion.

Questions:
Categorize each of the following as a process or an outcome criterion.

8. a. The client states he eats at least one food high in protein with each meal. Process?   Outcome?
   b. The nurse gives the client a list of foods high in protein. Process?   Outcome?
   c. The client walks at least one-half mile three times a week. Process?   Outcome?
   d. The nurse discusses the client's 180 heart rate during exercise as a measurement of the maximum desired stress on the heart. Process?   Outcome?

SUMMARY
Previously, only nursing actions have been evaluated with criteria. This focus on the nurse's actions excludes the client. Since the goal of nursing care is to promote optimal health for the client, it is essential to include the client in the evaluation of nursing care. An evaluation of a nurse's action must include both process and outcome criteria. Both types of criteria must be critical, single, observable, timed, and positive.

Questions:
9. a. Describe one nursing action you performed for a client in your last clinical experience.

© 1977 Wiley

b. Write one *process* criterion that evaluates your action above.

c. Write one *outcome* criterion that evaluates the client outcome from your action above.

GREAT! You have finished Activity 2. Now check your answers with those that follow. When you have answered all the questions successfully, you have completed Activity 2 of the module. Now continue to Activity 3, where you will apply the evaluation criteria in the complete evaluation process.

Answers

1. An evaluation criterion is a statement of a *critical condition* or *behavior.*
2. a. critical: thirty-pound weight loss shows important progress for an obese client
   b. noncritical: reading a magazine is not socializing with others and is not a critical factor showing progress for this client
   c. critical: knitting a blanket for an important occasion is important for this client with arthritis
3. a. no, there are two critical characteristics in the criterion
   b. "loss of thirty pounds in six weeks" or "loss of two inches at the waist in six weeks"
4. a. no, independent functioning is not an observable behavior itself
   b. "fed himself dinner without help after the tray is served" *or other* independent behaviors that are observable
5. a. no, it does not describe a specific time for the criterion to be met
   b. add any time which would be obtainable by that client (example: "the client states the correct schedule for his medications on the day of discharge from the hospital")
6. a. no, it is a negative characteristic
   b. any desirable behaviors such as: "all medications given in the exact dosage ordered by the physician"
7. f. any evaluation criterion related to understanding post operative care which is critical, single, observable, timed, and positive (example: "the client states to the nurse before discharge that he must elevate his leg above his waist for at least one hour each day for the following week")
8. a. outcome
   b. process
   c. outcome
   d. process
9. a. any nursing action
   b. a statement that describes a critical, single, observable, timed and positive behavior which is included in the nursing action
   c. a statement of evaluation criterion with the essential elements that describe a behavior that *results* from the nursing action

© 1977 Wiley

160 NURSING ASSESSMENT

ACTIVITY 3
ACTIONS IN THE EVALUATION PROCESS

Activity 3 describes the action in the evaluation process and guides the reader in applying the evaluation process to nursing actions. Complete the Activity by applying your clinical experiences and the evaluation concepts from the Activities you have completed so far.

THE EVALUATION PROCESS
The evaluation process is similar to the problem-solving process. Actually the evaluation process measures whether the problem was solved. It answers these questions: "Was a certain action performed in the desired manner?" "Was the desired outcome achieved?"

The evaluation process must include making an assessment, identifying goals, developing evaluation criteria, and comparing the actions to the criteria. The assessment and goals must focus on both the nurse and the client, just as the evaluation criteria focus on both.

Figure 1[8] shows the fundamental concepts of the evaluation process, which is composed of many interrelated actions; starts with an assessment phase; is based on specific evaluation criteria; focuses on both nurse actions and client outcomes; and is a continuous process with the result of one evaluation leading to the assessment phase of the next.

Questions:
Answer the following true or false. The evaluation process:

1. T   F   a.   uses general statements for evaluation
    T   F   b.   does not have to be considered until an action is performed
    T   F   c.   is one separate step in the problem-solving process
    T   F   d.   focuses mostly on the nurse's action
    T   F   e.   can be completed even if the nurse's goals are uncertain

APPLICATION OF THE EVALUATION PROCESS
Tim Bush, a new nurse in a cardiac care unit, used the evaluation process as a guide in developing his abilities for cardiac nursing. Tim performed the following actions in the evaluation process.

NURSE FOCUS   *CLIENT FOCUS*

I. ASSESSMENT

Determine Nurse's Abilities and Needs   *Determine Client's Abilities and Needs*

The nurse: The nurse:
—requested the staff nurse clinical competency   —observed the types of patients on the unit
  form from the unit supervisor.   and the type of care they needed.
—observed other nurses who were established   —recognized the patients needed close moni-
  on the unit to identify their usual nursing   toring of heart rhythms by the nurse.
  performances.
—recognized the new nurse's need to read electrocardiograms.

II. GOALS

Identify Nurse's Goals   *Identify Client's Goals*

—the nurse described the nursing goal as gain-   —the nurse recognized the client's goal of re-
  ing the ability to quickly read electrocardio-   ceiving immediate medical care following
  grams.   abnormal cardiac rhythms.

---
[8] Johnson, S. H., "The Evaluation in Nursing," 1976.

© 1977 Wiley

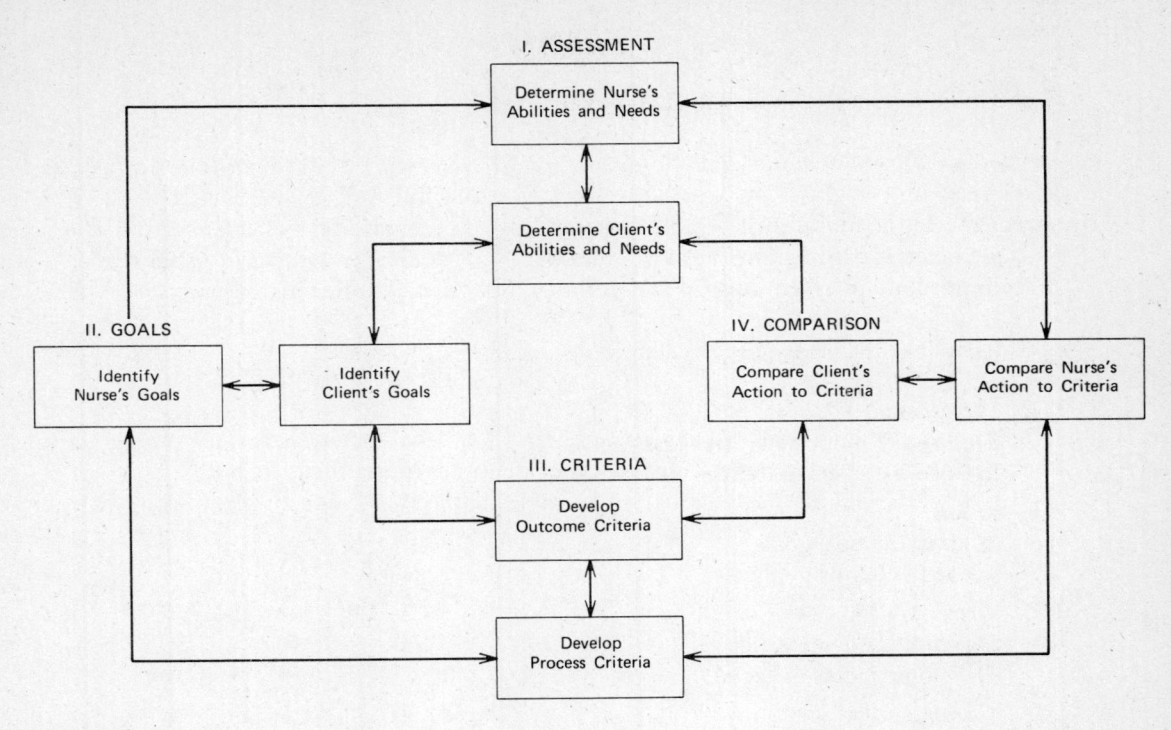

FIGURE 1
The evaluation process—a model.

III. CRITERIA

Develop Process Criteria

The nurse described the desired nursing performance with process criteria:
—within one week the nurse would attend a class on interpreting electrocardiograms.
—within one month the nurse would have identified all abnormal rhythms for the clients within ten seconds.

Develop Outcome Criteria

The nurse described the desired client outcome of her action:
—within the next month every client would have received cardiac intervention within twenty seconds after an abnormal heart pattern.

IV. COMPARISON

Compare Nurse Action to Criteria

The nurse:
—passed the test on interpreting electrocardiograms following the class.
—identified all four heart arrhythmias and summoned cardiac help within ten seconds.
—performed within the evaluation criteria.

Compare Client Action to Criteria

—The client received cardiac interventions within twenty seconds.
—For one arrhythmia the client received help after thirty seconds.
—The client outcome did not meet the evaluation criteria.

© 1977 Wiley

V. REASSESSMENT

This evaluation leads to the assessment again.

Determine Nurse's Abilities and Needs
The nurse:
—recognized the nurse must be able not only to read electrocardiograms but also to initiate immediate interventions for arrhythmias.

Determine Client's Abilities and Needs
The nurse:
—recognized the client's need for consistent medical treatment initiated immediately upon cardiac arrhythmia.

To review, the steps in the evaluation process are:

I. *Assessment*
   Determine nurse's abilities and needs
   Determine client's abilities and needs
II. *Goals*
   Identify nurse's goals
   Identify client's goals
III. *Criteria*
   Develop outcome criteria
   Develop process criteria
IV. *Comparison*
   Compare client's action to criteria
   Compare nurse's action to criteria

Question:
2. The nurse's activities in the left column below demonstrate some steps in the evaluation process. Match the nurse's activity with the step in the evaluation process.

   a. The client receives individual nursing care with precise actions that meet his personal style.
   b. The nurse recognizes that all of the clients have individual wishes and desires.
   c. The nurse identifies the goal to develop individualized care plans.
   d. The nurse describes what is desired: to complete a care plan that describes precise ways to care for the client for at least one day.

   I. *Assessment*—Determines abilities and needs of client and nurse.
   II. *Goals*—Identifies goals of client and nurse.
   III. *Criteria*—Develops criteria for client and nurse.
   IV. *Comparison*—Compares client and nurse action to criteria.
   V. *Reassessment*—Reassesses abilities and needs of client and nurse.

CONGRATULATIONS! After completing the activity and reviewing your answers, you have completed Activity 3. Go on to Activity 4.

Answers
1. a. F—these are very common false assumptions about evaluation
   b. F—they result in major difficulties in performance of evaluations
   c. F
   d. F
   e. F

© 1977 Wiley

2. a. IV, Comparison
   b. I or V, Assessment
   c. II, Goals
   d. III, Criteria

ACTIVITY 4
PLANNING AND PERFORMING THE EVALUATION

Activity 4 guides the reader in planning and performing the evaluation process in actual clinical practice.

ASSESSMENT STEP OF THE EVALUATION PROCESS
Complete each step in the evaluation process by recalling past clinical experiences and answering the questions.

Question:
1. a. List one nursing ability you need to refine.

   b. List one client need that would be met by your refinement of this skill.

GOAL STEP OF THE EVALUATION PROCESS

Question:
2. a. Identify your nursing goal in refining the ability mentioned above.

   b. Identify one client goal that would be reached by your refining the ability.

CRITERIA STEP OF THE EVALUATION PROCESS

Question:
3. a. Develop one process criterion that would be met by your refining the ability.

   b. Develop one outcome criterion that would demonstrate a desired outcome of the refinement of your ability.

COMPARISON STEP OF THE EVALUATION PROCESS

Question:
4. a. Carry out your nursing action and determine whether it met the process criterion above.
   b. Determine whether the outcome criterion was met with a desired outcome for your client.

© 1977 Wiley

REASSESSMENT STEP IN THE EVALUATION PROCESS

Question:
5. a. Based on whether you met the process criterion or not, reassess your nursing ability.

   b. Based on whether the client had the desired outcome or not, reassess the client's need for the refinement of your ability.

When you have answered the questions above and checked the answers, you have completed Activity 4.

CONGRATULATIONS! You have finished the last Activity of the module. Go on to the Posttest.

Answers
1. a. one nursing ability that needs to be refined
   b. one client need that would be met by the ability above
2. a. a nursing goal related to the ability above
   b. a client goal related to the nursing action above
3. a. process criterion that evaluates the nursing action
   b. outcome criterion that evaluates a client outcome
4. a. the action has or has not met the process criterion for the ability
   b. the action has or has not resulted in the desired outcome for the client
5. a. the nursing ability is still needed if the process criterion was not met; the nursing ability does not need to be refined if it met the process criterion
   b. the client still needs the nursing action if the outcome criterion was not met; the client does not still need the nursing action if the outcome criterion was met

POSTTEST

Complete the following questions in the spaces provided.

1. In one sentence define "evaluation process."

The following statements describe characteristics or values of the evaluation process. Answer each statement as True or False.

T F 2. The final goal of nursing evaluation is to determine if a nurse's performance meets acceptable criteria.

T F 3. Nursing evaluation influences future nursing performance.

T F 4. Evaluation is related to the Assessment part of the problem-solving process rather than the Problem Identification part.

T F 5. Nursing evaluation is performed after the nursing interventions have been performed.

T F 6. Citizens think the health team are adequately evaluating their own performance.

© 1977 Wiley

T F 7. Criteria that evaluate nursing care rather than medical care are easily developed.
T F 8. Continuing self-evaluation fosters positive feelings about evaluation.
T F 9. Evaluation encourages growth when it includes general areas of weakness rather than specific situations.
10. List three benefits you might receive from using peer evaluation of your nursing performance.

Three types of evaluation for the health team are listed below. Enter in the space provided the characteristic that best describes each type of evaluation.

_____ 11. utilization review
_____ 12. quality assurance
_____ 13. patient care audit

a. evaluation criteria include measures of optimum care
b. evaluates the use of health facilities
c. evaluates a client's health care over a period of time

Several evaluation criteria are listed below. Each criterion has at least one essential characteristic missing. State the missing characteristic and rewrite the criterion to include it.

14. Criterion: Three hours after admission the client has no difficulty breathing.
    Missing characteristic:
    Revised criterion:

15. Criterion: Before discharge the client states he will do a passive range of motion exercises to his leg three times a day and will drink 6 glasses of fluid per day.
    Missing characteristic:
    Revised criterion:

16. Criterion: The client correctly identified prescribed medications by sight.
    Missing characteristic:
    Revised criterion:

Demonstrate the planning and performance of the evaluation process by answering the questions on the clinical situation below. The evaluation will focus on the client.

Situation: As a new nurse in a community alcoholism project, you notice that five of the ten clients left the project in the first four weeks. The project calls for the client's involvement for eight weeks. You would like to evaluate the success of the new approaches you are taking.

17. *Assessment.* Describe what abilities and needs the clients have.

18. *Goals.* Identify one client goal related to the alcoholism project.

19. *Criteria.* Develop one outcome criterion for these clients.

Situation: In the situation above you tried several strategies. As a result, seven out of ten of the next group of clients stay in the program for four weeks. Six out of ten remain in the program to its completion and have had no liquor during or following the program. It is now two months since they completed the program.

© 1977 Wiley

166 NURSING ASSESSMENT

20. *Comparison.* Using the additional information above, compare the results of the nursing strategies by analyzing the results with your criterion.

GOOD! You have completed the Posttest. Check your answers. Each question is worth one point. You must have 17 points (85%) correct to pass the Posttest.

Answers

1. The evaluation process is a group of related *actions* that rate a *performance* based on specific *criteria.* (The italicized concepts must be present in the definition.)
2. F   3. T   4. F   5. F   6. F   7. F   8. T   9. F
10. increased self-worth, continued learning, increased stature related to peers, increased quality nursing performance (any three)
11. b. utilization review—evaluates the use of health facilities
12. a. quality assurance—evaluation criteria include measures of optimum care
13. c. patient care audit—evaluates a client's health care over a period of time
14. not positive (example of a revised criterion: three hours after admission the client's respirations were between 15-25 per minute)
15. not single characteristic (example of a revised criterion: before discharge the client states he will drink six glasses of fluid a day)
16. not timed (example of a revised criterion: on the day of discharge the client correctly identified prescribed medications by sight)
17. *assessment:* the clients need help against alcoholism and half of them need to remain in the program
18. *goal:* a client goal is to stop drinking or return to physical health
19. *criterion:* in the next group seven out of ten clients stay in the group. (any outcome criterion)
20. *comparison:* the results described in the situation meet or do not meet the criterion depending on the criterion developed in question 19

References

1. McClain, J. O., "Screening for Utilization Review," *American Journal of Public Health* 63 (1973): 247-251.
2. Tippett, J., "Developing a Utilization Review Model for Community Medical Health Centers," *Hospital and Community Psychiatry* 26 (1975): 165-166.
3. Maniaci, Marie, "Quality Assurance in the Provision of Hospital Care: Case Study," *Hospitals* 48 (1974): 81-83.
4. Eddy, Lyndall and Westbrook, Linda, "Multidisciplinary Retrospective Patient Care Audit," *American Journal of Nursing* 75 (1975): 961-963.
5. Orme, J. V., "Nurse Participation in Medical Peer Review," *Nursing Outlook* 22 (1974): 27-30.
6. Gold, H. et al., "Peer Review, A Working Experience," *Nursing Outlook* 21 (1973): 634-636.
7. Yura, Helen, *Guidelines for Review of Nursing Care at the Local Level,* American Nurses Association, 1976.
8. Johnson, S. H., "The Evaluation in Nursing," Class syllabus, 1976.

Suggested Readings

Flashner, B. A.; Reed, Shirley; Coburn, Robert; and Fine, Philip, "Professional Standards Review Organizations," *JAMA* 223 (1973): 1473–1484.

Keeler, J. D., "The Process of Program Evaluation," *Nursing Outlook* 20 (1972): 316–319.

Mayers, Marlene G., "A Search for Assessment Criteria," *Nursing Outlook* 20 (1972): 323–326.

Meleis, Afaf I. and Benner, Pat, "Process or Product Evaluation," *Nursing Outlook* 23 (1975): 303–307.

Shields, Mary, "An Evaluation Model for Service Programs," *Nursing Outlook* 22 (1974): 448–451.

Yura, Helen and Walsh, Mary, "Guidelines for Evaluation: Who, What, When, Where, and How?" *Supervisor Nurse* 3 (1972): 33–44.